Basic Health Care in Family Medicine and Public Health

Edited by Hülya Çakmur

Published in London, United Kingdom

Basic Health Care in Family Medicine and Public Health
http://dx.doi.org/10.5772/intechopen.1004496
Edited by Hülya Çakmur

Contributors
Darijana Antonić, Elizabeth Anne Lee, Faisal Abdullatif Alnaser, Hülya Çakmur, Jennifer Chiok Foong Loke, Kah Wai Lee, Slobodan Stanić, Takalani Edith Mutshatshi, Thabo Arthur Phukubye

Notice
Statements and opinions expressed in the chapters are these of the individual contributors and not necessarily those of the editors or publisher. No responsibility is accepted for the accuracy of information contained in the published chapters. The publisher assumes no responsibility for any damage or injury to persons or property arising out of the use of any materials, instructions, methods or ideas contained in the book.

First published in London, United Kingdom, 2025 by IntechOpen
IntechOpen is the global imprint of INTECHOPEN LIMITED, registered in England and Wales, registration number: 11086078, 167-169 Great Portland Street, London, W1W 5PF, United Kingdom

For EU product safety concerns: IN TECH d.o.o., Prolaz Marije Krucifikse Kozulić 3, 51000 Rijeka, Croatia, info@intechopen.com or visit our website at intechopen.com.

British Library Cataloguing-in-Publication Data
A catalogue record for this book is available from the British Library

Basic Health Care in Family Medicine and Public Health
Edited by Hülya Çakmur
p. cm.

This title is part of the Public Health Book Series, Volume 2
Series Editor: José Antonio Mirón Canelo

Print ISBN 978-1-83634-011-9
Online ISBN 978-1-83634-010-2
eBook (PDF) ISBN 978-1-83634-012-6
ISSN 3049-8872

If disposing of this product, please recycle the paper responsibly.

We are IntechOpen,
the world's leading publisher of
Open Access books
Built by scientists, for scientists

7,400+
Open access books available

193,000+
International authors and editors

210M+
Downloads

Our authors are among the

156
Countries delivered to

Top 1%
most cited scientists

12.2%
Contributors from top 500 universities

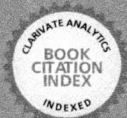

Interested in publishing with us?
Contact book.department@intechopen.com

Numbers displayed above are based on latest data collected.
For more information visit www.intechopen.com

IntechOpen Book Series
Public Health
Volume 2

Aims and Scope of the Series

Public health is what we as a society do collectively to contribute to and ensure the health and social conditions for the enjoyment of health as a resource for life. It can also be defined as science and research that promotes health, prevents disease, and improves populations' well-being and quality of life. Its objective is to know the risk factors that determine and condition the populations' health levels at present. At the end of the 20th century and the beginning of the 21st century, it is unjustifiable and regrettable that morbimortality according to age plays a leading role when the causes are mostly well known and therefore preventable, such as obesity, AIDS, cirrhosis, diabetes mellitus, addictions and cancer associated with the consumption of tobacco and alcohol, etc. In short, public health is science based on epidemiology and biostatistics, and currently, new technologies and artificial intelligence must be incorporated to identify patterns and trends in what we do collectively as a society to ensure living conditions and prevent risk factors that affect individual and population health. For all these reasons, it is essential to scientifically investigate and act on the determinants that impede the well-being and quality of life related to the health of people, patients, and populations in general, given that to control the determinants of diseases, it is important to control the environment and genetics. Consequently, the current fight for public health must prioritize the control of the environment, such as atmospheric and biological pollution and environmental and social biodiversity, promoting the sensitivity and training of society and its individuals by empowering them to make free and appropriate decisions about these aspects to lead healthy lifestyles based on motivation and responsibility in the face of the challenges they cope with from an individual point of view, such as dealing with the addictions that exist in today's complex world. Public health also requires an ethical vision and incorporates strategies to reduce social inequality.

Meet the Series Editor

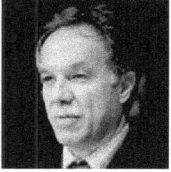

José Antonio Mirón Canelo is a physician, doctor, and professor of Preventive Medicine and Public Health at the Faculty of Medicine and Dentistry of the University of Salamanca with over 30 years of experience. He is the director of the USAL's Expert Degree in Health Management, currently in its 13th edition. Prof. Mirón Canelo directs a research group at the Research Institute of Biomedical Sciences (IBSAL) of the University of Salamanca focused on addressing the challenges and care needs of vulnerable people and patients such as the elderly with multiple pathologies and people with disabilities and dependence. As a teacher, he has been recognized for excellence in teaching three times in a period of five years.

Meet the Volume Editor

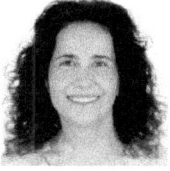

Hülya Çakmur graduated from the medical school at Atatürk University, Turkey. She completed her residency training in family medicine at Trakya University in Turkey and obtained a Ph.D. in Public Health from Dokuz Eylül University in Turkey. She has 26 years of practice experience as a specialist in family medicine, including 13 years of experience in public health as a Ph.D. prepared professional. She also studied sleep medicine at the University of Pittsburgh Medical Center in the USA and narrative medicine at St. Thomas University in Canada. Hülya Çakmur voluntarily studied geriatrics and published several studies in the field. She is an active member of the Turkish Medical Association and the European Academy of Teachers in General Practice/Family Medicine. She has 12 years of experience as a professor at the University of Kafkas in Turkey, where she is the Department of Family Medicine director. She has published more than thirty papers in reputed journals.

Contents

Preface

The primary task of the family physician is to ensure the implementation of basic health services. Family medicine centers are the places where basic health services meet the community. Family physicians must provide comprehensive, continuous and holistic health services to the registered population. Comprehensive health care focuses on finding the most appropriate solution by addressing both mental and physical, acute and chronic health problems of the individual together with the individual's family, the social environment to which the individual belongs and the country where the individual lives. For a health service to be called continuous, the physician must have prior knowledge of the individual at the client-physician meeting. The continuity of health records, space, and time is essential for continuous health care. Holistic health care is an approach that interprets health as a whole by evaluating the human being in all its dimensions. Family medicine's core competencies are managing primary (basic) health care services, person-centered care, community-oriented, unique problem-solving skills, comprehensive approach, and approach to the person as a bio-psycho-social whole. The family physician is responsible for the community's health and the effective use of resources and assumes a special responsibility for the community's health. The discipline of family medicine recognizes that it is responsible for the individual and society in health matters. It examines the patient's problems in the context of their social environment. The family physician should also be aware of the community's needs and collaborate with other sectors to find solutions to local health problems. Public health is another department that family physicians need to cooperate with in order to implement basic health services effectively. Public health is philosophically in agreement with basic health services. In other words, public health adopts the principles of basic health services, and even the reason for the existence of public health is to ensure the structuring of basic health services. Although it depends on societies' economic and social structure, effective and strong basic health services rely on the cooperation and joint productivity of family medicine and public health units.

Hülya Çakmur
Medical School,
Department of Family Medicine,
Kafkas University,
Kars, Turkey

Chapter 1

Introductory Chapter: Two Pillars of Basic Health Care – Family Medicine and Public Health

Hülya Çakmur

1. Introduction

Basic health care services are the universal preventive, promotive, curative and rehabilitative health care services that countries provide free of charge to the public on an equal basis and within their own economic means [1]. Health systems cover all health services, including disease prevention, health promotion, treatment when necessary, rehabilitation and palliative care. The main objective of basic health care services is to protect and improve health by making health services equally available and accessible to all segments of society. In order to achieve this goal, it is necessary to make appropriate investments in areas that form the basis of a healthy life, such as a livable clean environment, clean drinking water, easy access to healthy and safe food, a workplace and job security suitable for everyone's abilities, increasing social welfare and security, and retirement security [2]. These areas, which are defined within the scope of social determinants of health, are known as the main factors affecting health and well-being. These are the conditions in which we are born, grow, live, work and age. The effectiveness of basic health care services in the field of social determinants of health depends on the welfare of the society and the right health policies. Educational attainment, economic, cultural and family status affect health directly and indirectly. Poor social and economic conditions have a negative impact on health and can increase disease rates [1–3]. These conditions are often not the direct cause of disease but are described as the "cause of the causes" that lead to disease. In the area of social determinants of health in a society, the more accurate the investments mentioned above, from a clean environment to healthy food, the stronger the basic health services of the society. Although the main task of basic health care is preventive services, the implementation of these services is directly related to the economy of the country, as they also include outpatient treatment and rehabilitative services. Effective implementation of the health system depends on the knowledge, skills and motivation of health workers at the last step. However, in the first step, health policies need to be planned correctly [3].

2. Family medicine and public health

Family medicine and public health disciplines are the two supportive and executive bodies of basic health care in planning and implementation. These two disciplines can create a strong basic health care service by working together and in coordination with each other. It is clear that health protection can be achieved by fulfilling the social and economic determinants of health. Health promotion, on the other hand, is made possible by focusing on prevention and positively affecting the health and well-being of individuals and then societies. In other words, prosperous societies have healthy individuals and healthy individuals build prosperous societies [1]. The field of study of the public health discipline is the planning and supervision of social practices in the field of social determinants of health. Family medicine, on the other hand, is responsible for providing comprehensive integrated and continuous health care services that assume social responsibility as well as protecting and improving health on an individual basis. Health promotion is the process of enabling people to take responsibility for their health after countries have established the right health policies [4, 5]. Therefore, health promotion is the responsibility of both public health and family medicine disciplines. It is impossible to protect and improve health by focusing only on individual lifestyles. The mission of protecting and promoting health, which is the essence of basic health care, can be made possible by implementing the philosophy of public health through family medicine [6]. Health is an important economic sector. However, basic health care is inherently non-profit. Basic health care aims to make health care more accessible to those in need of care. Countries can determine the provision of these services according to their own medical needs and social welfare. The phenomenon of health protection and promotion is shaped and transformed according to scientific developments [7]. While combating the infectious diseases of the period was the key task of basic health care services in the historical process, gradually, combating metabolic and malignant diseases and even anti-aging practices can almost be included in the scope of basic health care services. Therefore, basic health care services are not concrete services with strictly defined boundaries, but rather services that are redefined according to the needs of the period, but whose philosophy remains the same [4, 5, 7].

The principles of basic health care can be summarized in four points:

1. Equality: The principle of equity argues that health is an inherent human right and should be provided equally and fairly to everyone in society, not only to those who can afford it. The applicability of this principle is directly related to social and economic welfare [1–3].

2. Self-responsibility: Each individual should know the value of his/her own health and be responsible for his/her health. For this purpose, individuals should be educated about health, and healthy behavior patterns should be acquired at an early age. The applicability of this principle is directly related to family medicine services. In comprehensive and continuous family medicine services, each individual-physician encounter should be considered an educational opportunity, and health education should be provided in accordance with the needs of the individual [1–3].

3. Coordination of health services: Considering the social, economic, cultural and social determinants of health, it is clear that health cannot be limited to the medical dimension alone. Therefore, coordination with all sectors in the society is necessary [1–3].

4. International solidarity: A health problem in one part of the world affects the whole world in a very short time. Therefore, health is a world and human problem [1–3].

For optimal delivery of primary health care:

- The community should participate in health services.

- Health services should be provided in a team approach.

- Units should be established for the first application.

- Health service units should be integrated.

- Preventive, curative, rehabilitative and health promotion services should be considered as a whole.

- Services must be continuous [1–3].

3. Conclusion

The disciplines of public health and family medicine, which constitute the planning, supervision and implementation parts of basic health care services, should act together to prevent and eliminate factors that adversely affect health. Health services cannot be considered independent from the economy at every level. In order to plan and implement optimum basic health care services in accordance with the changing basic health needs of the society according to the age we live in, the economic and social welfare of the society is necessary.

Author details

Hülya Çakmur
Head of Family Medicine Department, Kafkas University, Turkey

*Address all correspondence to: hulyacakmur@gmail.com

IntechOpen

References

[1] Eddy DM. What care is 'essential'?
What services are 'basic'? Journal of
the American Medical Association.
1991;**265**(6):782, 786-788. DOI: 10.1001/
jama.265.6.782

[2] Öztek Z. Temel Sağlık Hizmetleri.
1978-2018. Available from: http://www.
hasuder.org.tr

[3] WHO The World Health Report 2008:
Primary Health Care now More Than
Ever. ISBN 978 92 4 156373. Available
from: http://www.who.int/whr/2008/en/
index.html

[4] Tulchinsky T, H, Varavikova EA.
Chapter 6 - family health. In:
The New Public Health. 3rd ed.
2014. pp. 311-379. DOI: 10.1016/
B978-0-12-415766-8.00006-9

[5] Tulchinsky TH, Varavikova EA.
Chapter 10 - Organization of Public
Health Systems. In: The New Public
Health. 3rd ed. 2014. pp. 535-
573. DOI: 10.1016/
B978-0-12-415766-8.00010-0

[6] "Health Promotion is the Process
of Enabling People to Increase
Control Over, and to Improve
Their Health." Health Promotion
Glossary. 1998. Available from:
https://www.who.int/health-topics/
health-promotion#tab=tab_1

[7] Stanimirović D, Pribaković BR.
Human resource planning in health
care: Outlining a basic model and
related complexities. Studies in
Health Technology and Informatics.
2022;**299**:279-282. DOI: 10.3233/
SHTI220999

Chapter 2

Primary Health Care Is the Foundation of Health Services

Faisal Abdullatif Alnaser

Abstract

Primary healthcare (PHC) is a fundamental type of health service considered the foundation of the health service pyramid. It entails providing continuous personal and comprehensive health services, including preventive and curative health services. Studies worldwide reported that PHC is an efficient, cost-effective service that helps upgrade the health of the person, their family, and the community.

Keywords: family medicine, primary healthcare, family physician, patient-centered care, continuity of care, health for all, community participation

1. Introduction

This chapter will provide an overview of primary healthcare (PHC) and family medicine. It will begin by defining them, and then it will delve into the historical perspectives of their origin and the development that happened with time in order to establish themselves professionally and academically. The significance and value of such services are later discussed, along with the strategy employed to ensure that everyone in the community has access to healthcare. More details will be shed on their pillars, including prevention, health promotion, risk reduction, a holistic approach, and person-centered healthcare as opposed to disease-focused healthcare. More details will be provided about how affordable, cost-effective, and efficient it is as a means of delivering healthcare, with an emphasis on equity, community engagement, and intersectoral collaboration. Additionally, the chapter will demonstrate how PHC can provide the best healthcare possible to everyone, fulfilling the slogan of a family doctor for every family while supporting community-based health needs and initiatives. At the end of the chapter, the barriers and challenges that stand in the way of its full implementation are also highlighted.

2. Body of the manuscript

2.1 Primary healthcare (PHC)

Healthy living is defined as a life free from illness and characterized by good social, mental, and physical well-being for each individual and every community. To do that, a comprehensive health service that provides sickness prevention, treatment,

IntechOpen

rehabilitation, and palliative care must be provided using a holistic approach. Each such component is specified in the PHC tenets. PHC is a kind of healthcare service that focuses on maintaining and restoring people's general well-being by identifying health problems and offering treatment at the earliest stages of illness development. Furthermore, PHC emphasizes continuous medical care that is personalized, within the family context, and person-centered as opposed to disease-centered. It is a very cost-effective way of providing healthcare services while maintaining intersectoral cooperation, population equity, and community engagement to respond to community-based health needs initiatives.

The World Health Organization (WHO) views PHC as a cornerstone of medical service that is critical for promoting health. WHO publication, "Primary Health Care: Now More Than Ever," highlights the value of PHC. It suggests that PHC reforms would work toward achieving social protection and universal access, enhancing health equity, rearranging service delivery to better meet the needs and expectations of the public, securing healthier communities through improved public policies, and reorganizing health leadership around more efficient government and engaging key stakeholders. A PHC program must be easily accessible to the general public, and its technology and procedures must be accepted by society for it to be successful [1–7]. According to various reports, it is critical to maintain PHC as the initial point of contact of the public with the healthcare system. Without effective primary care that can meet the needs and ambitions of the population's health, the health systems will not be able to withstand challenges [8]. Successful PHC services require the active participation of the community, non-profit organizations, the private sector, and the health ministries to guarantee that everyone in the community receives the finest healthcare available, leading to general improvement in the population's health.

Reports have indicated that strengthening PHC as the first point of contact with the health system is critical. Without effective primary care that can meet the needs of the population's health and ambitions for overall well-being, the health systems of the future will not be able to withstand challenges [8].

PHC is the foundation of the pyramidal health services offered to the population, which could collapse without a solid. It plays a major role in every sector of health, especially public health, and community, and the best example was the vital role PHC played in overcoming the late COVID-19 pandemic in 2019 and limiting its withdrawal effects. However, the tale was not so promising in countries where PHC was not very well developed. Dr. Tedros Adhanom Ghebreyesus, the WHO Director-General, stated "*We have seen during the pandemic that the poor, the most vulnerable, and the most marginalized people paid the highest cost. Equity cannot and must not wait. WHO is committed to working with governments, international financing institutions, partners, young people, and civil society to radically change course through prioritizing action and investments into a primary health care approach*" [9].

2.2 Family medicine (FM) and family physician (FP)

The recognition of FM as a relatively young topic in medical specializations has increased during the last three to four decades. Every country's health system is presumed to be supported by the clinical and academic areas of FM [10]. FM is considered to be the only medical discipline that focuses on meeting the needs of individuals, families, and communities. With the emphasis on the family as the unit of care to offer PHC services, FPs receive specialized training, enabling them to provide high-quality healthcare to patients of all ages [11]. FM which offers a very cost-effective, acceptable, and efficient, leads with no doubt to the improvement of the health standard of the individual and the whole nations, particularly in developing countries [12, 13].

FPs are general practitioners who possess the necessary credentials, education, and expertise to provide optimal PHC services. They are highly skilled doctors who are knowledgeable about contemporary science and technology, allowing them to provide screening services, early diagnosis, preventative care, and treatment [14]. Because FPs handle a lot of ambiguous and undifferentiated problems that are presented in the early stages of disease development, they operate in an environment where diagnostic uncertainty is higher. Regardless of age, sex, religion, or beliefs, they provide medical, psychological, and social care to all members of the family. FPs are well-versed in considering a variety of other factors that may impact a person's health when assessing their condition, including the family's lifestyle, beliefs, and practices; the dynamics within the family; the neighborhood's influence; the community's factors; and the impact of the society in which they live. Not to mention keeping in mind other significant elements like people's occupation, race, religion, and customs. Because of this, the FPs' obligations for a person's health take into account the framework of a variety of individual, family, and community issues, in addition to the person's mind and spirit. FPs' main responsibilities include promoting health, health education, providing preventative care, treating both acute and chronic illnesses, and relieving any physical or psychological effects that may arise from an Illness [15]. Because of their close relationship with family members, FPs are expected to serve as the primary medical advisors to the entire family on any health and psychosocial issues. This is because FPs are uniquely qualified to understand the factors and other circumstances that contribute to a patient's suffering, as well as the potential emotional and psychosocial repercussions for both the patient and their family. FPs are regarded as leaders in their field and are guardians, champions, and protectors of the patient's and family's safety throughout any health issue [16]. As a result, FPs are truly comprehensive physicians whose care is not only restricted to a single organ but offers overall care for all individuals, from the moment of birth until the end of life. This is what distinguishes FPs from several other specialties.

In addition to enhancing health and raising the standard of treatment, the FPs' responsibilities initiatives will assist in reducing the financial toll that an illness may take on individuals, their families, the community, and ultimately the government. Therefore, full adoption of FM's slogan, "a family physician for each family," is the perfect way to improve health and raise the health bar in any nation [17]. Thus, governments, insurance companies, and members of various social classes (especially those from lower and middle socioeconomic classes) benefit from the effective implementation of PHC. Ultimately by fortifying PHC, the government may focus on repairing other facilities and raising the standard of public health in general.

2.3 Family medicine and primary healthcare's historical perspective

The development of PHC/FM over the past century was prompted by several factors that have impacted the population's health. For example, PHC/FM was introduced as a substitute for general practice to counteract the decline in the role of traditional general practitioner since the year 1900 and to address the fragmentation of the current medical field into far too many small specialties and subspecialties as a result of significant advancements in medical technology; in response to the loss of continuity and comprehensiveness of care, to address the change in care that has occurred from a person-centered to a disease-centered approach, to include additional critical elements, such as social and psychological aspects, which are vital either in the course of the illness or as a result of it, and, in addition, PHC/FM was created in response to the growing dissatisfaction with the healthcare model and the necessity for developing an ideal model while caring for a sick person [18–20].

Having said that, PHC is not a novel idea; it has been around for a while and has been used in the past. During their profession, Avicenna, Alrazi, Al-Zahrawi, and other early Muslim physicians strongly embraced FM and the PHC system during their practice [21, 22]. They were holistic medical practitioners who considered the body as well as the soul. As a result, they went by the name Alhakeem, or the Wiseman because most of those scholars were experts in many other scientific domains and philosophers in addition to their medical specialization.

Although many of the concepts of FM as a distinct specialty did not exist at the time, Muslim physicians made several significant contributions that encompassed the concepts of comprehensive, patient-centered care. During their practice, they utilized all of the main FM and PHC components, including:

- Comprehensive care: looking at the ill patient as a human being who needs physical and spiritual care [23].

- Community-based and diverse patient population care: Ancient Muslim doctors never rejected any patients based on factors related to their roots, origin, religion, or beliefs. They took care of their patients and visited them at home regardless of whether they were wealthy or impoverished and lived in cities or rural areas [24–27].

- Dietary interventions: Al-Razi used to fortify his treatment regimen for an illness with advice on a healthy diet and nutrition [21].

- Prevention and continuity of care: They believed in prevention and continuity of care as an important way of maintaining health.

- General practice: Many of them were generalists with expertise in many medical specialties. Also, they applied the concept of evidence-based medicine during their practice by documenting patients' medical histories and clinical observations [28–30]

- Patient education: Almost all scholars have authored many medical textbooks addressing most of the illnesses that affect various organs in the body and other books on general health education. Al-Razi, who was considered the father of psychology and psychotherapy, wrote many books, one of which was a do-at-home book that illustrated medical advice for the general public [23, 28, 29, 31]. The "AL qanoon fe al tibb" which was a textbook of medicine, was written by Avicenna [23, 32]. Al-Zahrawi, who contributed to the development of ophthalmology, was a prolific writer on medical subjects and the inventor of various surgical devices. The Prophet Muhammad's female companion Rufaydah al-Aslamiyya is credited with creating what may have been the first transportable medical tent for patient treatment—an early example of community-based medical care [29, 33–35]. Moreover, to learn and teach others, many of those scholars translated the Greek and Roman medical textbooks into Arabic, used them during their medical breakthroughs, and provided them as a source of medical education references for the next generation of practitioners [23].

PHC has been proposed since the turn of the century as a name to replace other general healthcare services with a concept that focuses on the individual and the community. The concept of PHC was first proposed by the WHO Executive Council via a study done in January 1975. The study outlined seven principles that governments and health authorities should follow to improve the quality of healthcare: [36].

1. *Providing healthcare that is easily accessible in the community*

2. *Involving local communities in health efforts*

3. *Optimizing local community resilience to health issues*

4. *Ensuring the availability of health-promotive, preventive, and curative efforts in a health service*

5. *Providing human resources who are trained to provide health services closest to the community*

6. *Providing an environment that supports health efforts closest to the community*

7. *Integrating public healthcare with other sectors of life.*

But it was not until 1978 that the Alma Ata Conference on PHC in Kazakhstan rang the bell for international attention. A total of 134 nations unanimously agreed on a resolution declaring the need for coordinated efforts to address the social, economic, and political causes of ill health. The concept of "health for all by the year 2000" was eventually agreed upon as the primary principle aiming to develop a healthy society in member countries. This marked the first time that the world acknowledged inequalities in access to health care. Hence, the health policy of most nations around the globe was greatly impacted by the Alma-Ata Declaration, which expanded the definition of health to include social determinants and social justice in addition to medical measures [37].

The following were the declaration's main points [37–42].

The Alma-Ata Declaration highlights the disparity in access to healthcare between individuals in developing and underdeveloped nations. It emphasizes the need to address the social, political, and economic implications of this inequality and stresses the importance of closing this gap. The declaration views global health as a matter of social justice and calls for collaboration between governments and social organizations to find solutions.

The declaration affirms the right of every individual to participate in decisions regarding their healthcare, regardless of their location, and commits nations under the WHO to ensure access to quality and affordable healthcare. Moreover, it underscores the importance of primary healthcare through practical, scientific, and socially acceptable methods to promote the overall well-being of individuals worldwide.

The Alma-Ata Declaration sets the target year of 2020 for nations to reallocate a significant portion of their military budgets toward healthcare for their citizens. These are ambitious objectives for both developing and underdeveloped nations, which continue to face challenges in achieving them due to internal and external conflicts.

Following the Alma Ata Declaration, Canada ratified the Ottawa Charter for Health Promotion in 1986, which stated: "*To achieve health for all, and to reach a state of complete physical, mental, and social well-being, people are expected to be able to recognize health issues, must be able to identify and realize aspirations, satisfy needs, and change or cope with the environment.*" The Charter continues to be an essential guide for the implementation of health promotion [43].

On the thirtieth anniversary of the 2008 Alma Ata Declaration, the WHO published a paper titled "Primary Health Care: Now More Than Ever," urging advancements in the field of medicine. It stipulates four key points, which are: *first, accessible health care services, where the governments have to ensure that everybody, regardless of personal or financial circumstances, has access to the available health facilities; second, every member of society must attain a state of mental, bodily, or social health in addition to raising the caliber of medical equipment and/or human resources; third, putting more accountability on people in charge of healthcare management, in which the governments need to ensure that all health service providers lay out equal access to all members of society without exception; and finally, enable public policies that safeguard and advance public health. Countries must promote suitable public policies and public health services while preserving the spirit of equality and human rights* [44].

Two years after the first report, the WHO released a second one entitled "Health System Financing: The Path to Universal Coverage." It emphasized the idea of Universal Health Coverage (UHC), which is a health service system that safeguards the public and ensures equal access to high-quality medical treatment without financial constraints. The progress of FM globally was aided by such an idea [45]. Therefore FM was able to contribute to the restoration of continuity of care and doctor-patient interaction, which the growing specializations had undermined [18]. Such a move has also assisted in enhancing rural healthcare by motivating doctors to work in underprivileged areas [20].

In 2018, a second international conference on the value of basic healthcare was held in Astana, Kazakhstan. It emphasized the vital role of PHC worldwide. The proclamation seeks to guarantee everyone, wherever they are, to gain the benefit of the best attainable standard of health by ensuring excellent PHC. Again, the adoption of the Astana Declaration highlighted the importance of PHC in accomplishing both the Sustainable Development Goals and UHC [46, 47]. It underlined that the PHC strategy should be considered the most practical means of resolving the present problems with health and the health system sustainably [48]. Moreover, it highlighted the importance of political commitment from governmental organizations, non-governmental bodies, professional associations, academic institutions, and international agencies to PHC implementation [47].

2.4 Family medicine training programs and academic departments

Since FM was considered as a separate specialty in the middle of the 20th century, there was a need to meet the requirement for the production of highly qualified primary care physicians who could provide patients and families with comprehensive, ongoing care within the framework of their communities. For that, it was necessary to develop formal and standard-based education and training in PHC [18], which incorporated a comprehensive program that included health maintenance, promotion, and prevention for individuals as well as their families.

The following worldwide initiatives were made to academize the training in FM since the formal foundation of the specialty in the 1960s; [19].

- In 1947, the American Academy of General Practice was founded, which later, in 1971, renamed itself the American Academy of Family Physicians Academy [18]. This has played a major role in the recognition of the specialty.

- In 1964, the American Medical Association Council on Medical Education appointed an Ad Hoc Committee on Education for Family Practice. The committee issued its report entitled "Meeting the Challenge of Family Practice" which structured the FM curriculum and the training program [49]. These initiatives were granted financial and technical support by federal legislation in the late 1960s and early 1970s, which further accelerated the discipline's growth [50, 51].

- In 1969, FM in the USA was approved as a new specialty and a 3-year residency program in family medicine was structured and FM residency programs started having a significant impact on PHC services [52].

- In 1971, the American Board of Family Practice (ABFP) became the twentieth medical specialty board [53].

- In 1966, the United Kingdom introduced FM training programs, for the first time. Subsequently, and during the same decade, comparable initiatives were launched in Canada.

- By 1977, family medicine departments had become popular. While academic departments, divisions, and residency programs were present in almost all US medical schools. This move contributed to the specialty's institutionalization [50, 53].

- Family medicine residency programs (FPRP) grew quickly, from 30 in 1969 to 219 programs by 1975 in the USA [50]. More countries around the world started laying the foundation for FPRP. Studies showed that the number of countries that started the residency program increased within 20 years from 56 to 132 countries (between 1995 and 2015) [3, 10].

- Over the past few decades, FPRP programs have spread quickly to the majority of countries worldwide, although implementation models, types of training, standards, and recognition vary greatly from country to country based on each country's context and health system. In line with the recommendation from the World Health Organization for comprehensive, person-centered, first-contact, and community-based generalist medical care, FPRP laid the groundwork for holistic patient-centered healthcare [45].

- In 1980, the Kingdom of Bahrain and the Republic of Lebanon launched the first FPRP in the Arab world. It was a three-year training program, which was increased to 4 years after some time. Subsequently, many more Arab nations took that initiative.

- In 1978, the Council of the Arab Health Ministers (A division from the Arab League) decided to create the "Arab Board of Health Specializations (ABHS)" with its headquarters in Damascus, Syria. ABHS's main goal was to work on raising the level of medical science and practice in the Arab world so that health services are improved. To assist and encourage the Arab nations in creating and establishing FM services and initiating FPRP programs, the Family Medicine Council within the Arab Board was founded in 1985. It assumed responsibility for helping Arab nations to establish FM discipline, initiate and accredit existing FPRP programs and was accountable for graduating competent FP specialists by offering end-of-program standardized examinations. The program's curriculum, in addition to training in various medical disciplines, contained preventative care, behavioral health, and community medicine modules [18]. The first batch of Arab board-certified FPs graduated in 1990 [54].

- More countries in the Middle East region have started initiating FM training programs. The sequence was as follows: in Turkey, it started in 1961, Bahrain and Lebanon in 1979, Jordan in 1981, Kuwait in 1983, Saudi Arabia in 1987, Qatar and the United Arab Emirates in 1994, Oman in 1994, Iraq in 1996, Egypt in 2003, Iran in 2005, Libya and Syria in 2006, Palestine and Sudan in 2010, Tunisia in 2011, Morocco in 2023, and Yemen and the rest of the countries to start [55, 56].

- Moreover, universities in the Arab countries began establishing separate departments for family medicine [55, 57]. With the establishment of FM as a separate specialty, primary care physicians' education and requirements were codified and academized [18, 50].

2.5 Why are family medicine and primary health care so crucial?

PHC services supervised by FPs offer a variety of high-quality, easily accessible healthcare services. Because FPs started gaining a good reputation worldwide for providing efficient health services, many countries around the world started implementing FM programs and changing their health centers' structures and policies to adopt such a concept. In Canada, it is notable to state that, 70% of the Canadian healthcare services are provided by FPs. There is ample evidence connecting FPs to improved health outcomes, reduced costs, greater health equity, and a critical role in protecting and enhancing population health [45, 58, 59]. FPs also play a significant part in enhancing patient outcomes, reducing mortality rates, and cutting down on ER visits, hospital stays, and healthcare expenditures [60]. PHC is designed to function in both daily and emergency scenarios. It has been demonstrated that it substantially reduced the COVID-19 pandemic's detrimental effects on the healthcare system and to a large extent it helped in controlling both the spread of the virus and its aftereffects.

2.5.1 Better health indicators and outcomes

The introduction of FM services, which are provided by FPs, has generally improved health indicators in numerous countries. In the USA, studies showed that people who receive care from PHC physicians (in the USA, besides FPs, they also include general internal medicine or general pediatric doctors) are healthier, and those US states with higher ratios of primary care physicians in the population had better health outcomes. Studies found that FP supply was substantially correlated with lower all-cause mortality (which included mortality from heart disease, cancer, or stroke; infant mortality; low birth weight; and poor self-reported health.) in the USA between 1985 and 1995, whereas an increase in specialty physicians was linked to a higher death rate [61–63].

Studies conducted in the UK, where FP is known as a general practitioner (GP), revealed that each additional GP per 10,000 population (a 15 to 20% increase) is significantly associated with about a 6% decrease in mortality and a decrease in hospital admission rates by about 14 per 100,000 for acute illnesses and about 11 per 100,000 for chronic illnesses [64]. In addition, the ratio of GPs to the population was significantly associated with lower all-cause mortality, acute myocardial infarction mortality, avoidable mortality, acute hospital admissions for both chronic and acute conditions, and teenage pregnancies [65, 66]. Similarly, a study from Canada reported that every additional 10 FPs per 100,000 population will result in 15 fewer deaths, 40 fewer hospitalizations, and an average increase in life expectancy of 52 days [60]. According to a Brazilian study, implementing FM lowered the infant mortality rate from 21 per 1000 live births to 7 per 1000 over 2 years [67]. A Swedish study indicated that having a doctor in the family decreased other family members' mortality by 10%. In Turkey, however, significant progress was made in immunization, mobile health services, and patient follow-up for expectant mothers and infants after family medicine was introduced. Families led by health professionals have been found to have a lower prevalence of chronic illnesses, and FM offers better outcomes for managing chronic conditions [17, 68–72]. FPs provide patients with comprehensive, continuous, coordinated, affordable, and convenient care that can improve health outcomes. The higher proportion of primary care doctors in the general population was said to be the reason behind better preventive care, fewer hospitalization rates, and significantly lower overall healthcare costs compared to other specialties [65]. FPs can provide better care and improve the patient's and family's health standards by maintaining continuity of care. The longer the relationship between the FP and the family, the greater the decrease in hospital admissions, visits to the emergency department, and the rate of mortality [59, 73, 74].

2.5.2 In terms of money saving

Studies have shown that FM has a major economic benefit by reducing pointless doctor visits and/or hospital stays [17, 70, 74, 75]. Because FPs are trained to deal with the majority of clinical and emergency cases, fewer referrals to specialists are made, which lowers the overall cost of delivering healthcare. Research revealed a statistically significant correlation between family medicine certification and low referral rates [76]. Furthermore, the majority of FPs are capable of carrying out simple surgical procedures, which lowers the expense of healthcare services by avoiding the need to refer patients with such needs to secondary healthcare providers. A Stanford University study found that a family doctor performing minor procedures saved 70% of the cost of each treatment—that is, $551 on average—when compared to specialized care. Consequently, there is compelling evidence associating cost savings with comprehensive care, which is the principal responsibility of FPs [71, 77–80].

2.5.3 Patient satisfaction

Due to increased doctor-patient interactions, longer consultation times, continuity of care, and improved accessibility, it has been discovered that the provision of FM services is associated with higher patient satisfaction [72]. Families are also happier because the majority of their needs for health services can be met by a nearby accessible health centre that offers a range of excellent medical services in one convenient location [81].

2.5.4 Comprehensive care

Within FM, there is a compassionate policy that addresses the physical, mental, and social facets of health rather than concentrating just on treating particular symptoms [73, 82]. Studies demonstrated that this tactic will greatly improve health outcomes. Furthermore, by integrating preventive care, health could be preserved by using routine exams to spot potential health problems as early as possible [81].

2.6 Challenges to PHC

Although 90% of people in any society need PHC, according to the WHO and other international health organizations, it is disappointing to learn that, this new field initially ran into financial difficulties and only 10% of the health budget in most countries is allocated to PHC. Though numerous studies have suggested that PHC and FM may be the solution to the majority of medical and psychosocial health issues furthermore, WHO indicates that two billion people experience severe financial hardship as a result of healthcare costs and that over half of the world's population still lacks access to basic health services.

While FPs are capable of dealing with a wide range of medical disorders, treating patients of all ages, caring for the entire family, from young children to senior citizens, and offering exceptional services to improve the health of individuals and the community, the main challenge remains the shortage in their number. If this problem is not addressed, the quality of PHC services will be severely compromised, and ultimately, the population's overall health will be affected [60, 73, 82, 83]. Problems with professional practice, professional development, knowledge, and resistance from other specialists are among the other most significant challenges to PHC.

- Lack of funding, inadequate PHC infrastructure, and a shortage of medical personnel and supplies are some of the biggest issues facing PHC in developing nations [8].

- With fewer academic teachers dedicated to teaching undergraduate students, FM is still an unfinished field, knowledge and professional development are challenged by this factor. Additionally, the organizational, conceptual, and methodological content of FM is less well-defined, which contributes to the barriers that young physicians face when considering careers in this field.

- The following summarizes the main barriers and difficulties that PHC implementation faces:

- Lack of a developed infrastructure: Many medical schools lack the departments, faculty, and curriculum required to support their training initiatives because FM is still a relatively new field [18, 84].

- Requirements for changes in health policies: FM faces obstacles against its full implementation because of the need for a significant change in health management and policies. Therefore, a comprehensive vision and strong leadership qualities with commitment to PHC implementation should be reflected in the political decisions, leadership, and governance that accompany it [85].

- Limited awareness: Lack of understanding about the role of family medicine and how effective it is, may be the reason for why many policymakers remain unconvinced in the field [18, 57].

- Limited resources: Many low- and middle-income nations lack the necessary funds to set up an ideal PHC properly. While, to globally scale up the PHC approach in low- and middle-income countries, the WHO declared that an additional investment of at least US$ 200–328 billion per year, or roughly 3.3% of the national gross domestic product, is necessary. In a few other countries, PHC, family medicine departments, and programs are not adequately funded by health providers or academic institutions [9, 18].

- Poor Infrastructural Capacity: It is notable that in many countries, the buildings of the PHC center and its facilities are less attractive than the secondary or tertiary care facilities and lack important diagnostic and management equipment. Furnishing the PHC setup with the required up-to-date technology, digitalization, and computerization are challenges that work against the full expansion of the PHC's scope.

- Lack of the community's understanding and education about PHC.

- Ambiguity about the roles and responsibilities of FM: The identity of the discipline is still unclear, particularly concerning training, the majority of which takes place in hospitals or tertiary care units [18, 84]. It is challenging for the training program to teach and train physicians in a range of subjects and clinical cases while maintaining their level of proficiency when it takes place only in a PHC facility [86].

- The need for a dynamic curriculum: To address the comprehensive, continuous care model of family medicine, a new regularly updated curriculum should be developed [84].

- Lack of qualified faculty: Compared to other specialties, FM has fewer qualified FM consultants and well-trained teachers which could impact the quality of residents' supervision [84]. Moreover, the shortage of FP consultants is mostly related to income as both the income and the prestige for other specialties are higher in many countries. Therefore, occasionally, it is challenging to attract medical students to PHC.

- The global supply of FPs is still limited, particularly in developing nations: Many studies have shown the shortage in the ratio of FPs to the population. In South Africa (both in the public and private sectors), in 2015, there were only 0.1 family doctors per 10,000 people. By comparison, this figure was 0.2 in Brazil and 1.2 in China [87, 88]. One of the primary causes of this shortage is the fact that FPs often earn less money than their colleagues, who are specialists and do not have as glamorous a job as the others.

- Inadequate and ineffective referral mechanisms between PHC and secondary or tertiary care: A two-way referral system is necessary for an effective health system and to improve population health standards. The first step involves sending patients from the PHC facilities to specialized care for advice, additional management, or consultation, and the second is receiving feedback from the specialist to support the PHC provider's ongoing medical education and aid in the patient's continuity of care. A referral system should be well-developed that will be backed up by the most recent advancements in communication technology, and transparent, with a strong monitoring system.

- Opposition from other specialties: Certain well-established medical specialties oppose family medicine because of either a conflict of interest or a misunderstanding of its purpose and goals [18].

- Difficulty in implementing person-centered care rather than disease-centered care: It requires skill and experience to practice person-centered care. Moreover, the shortfall of the time allocated for every PHC consultation hinders the FP from reaching that goal [6, 7, 89].

- Burnout: FPs often face high levels of burnout due to increased workload, long working hours, and administrative burdens.

- Ambiguity and complexity of case presentation: It is challenging for some care providers when they work with uncertainty.

- Insufficient prospects for PHC employees to advance their education, receive CPD, or advance in their careers.

- Lack of social and community involvement: Leading to separation between the services offered and the community needs.

Finally, it is encouraging to state that most of the aforementioned problems are being gradually and progressively resolved as a result of a greater awareness of PHC's benefits in many nations. It is crucial to understand that all the obstacles and difficulties must be resolved if the choice is made to have a fully functional, effective PHC system.

Nomenclature

PHC	primary health care
FM	family medicine
FP	family physician
UHC	universal health coverage
CPD	continuous professional education
WHO	World Health Organization
GP	general practitioner
ABFM	American board of family practice
FPRP	family practice residency training programs
ABHS	Arab board of health specializations

Author details

Faisal Abdullatif Alnaser[1,2,3,4]

1 Department of Primary Health Care and Public Health, Imperial College, London, UK

2 WONCA EMR (World Congress for Family Physicians), Belgium

3 Bahrain Family Physician Association, Bahrain

4 Home Health Care Centre, Bahrain

*Address all correspondence to: falatf@gmail.com

IntechOpen

References

[1] World Health Organization. The World Health Report 2008: Primary Care (now more than ever). Available from: http://www.who.int/whr/2008/en/ [Accessed: October, 2017]

[2] World Health Organization. Global Strategy on Human Resources for Health: Workforce 2030. Available from: http://www.who.int/hrh/resources/pub_globstrathrh-2030/en/

[3] World Health Organization. Social Determinants of Health. 2006. Available from: https://www.who.int/teams/social-determinants-of-health/declaration-of-alma-ata

[4] Faisal Abdullatif Alnaser. Primary health care: The foundation of the health system. International Journal of Family Medicine and Primary Care. 2021;2(2):1-4

[5] van Weel C, Alnasir F, Farahat T, Usta J, Osman M, Abdulmalik M, et al. Primary healthcare policy implementation in the Eastern Mediterranean region: Experiences of six countries. European Journal of General Practice. 2018;24(1):39-44

[6] Alnasir F, Jaradat A. Patient-centered care; physicians view of obstacles against and ideas for implementation. International Journal of Medical Research & Health Sciences. 2016;5(4):161-168

[7] Qidwai W, Nanji K, Khoja TAM, Rawaf S, AlKurashi NY, Alnasir F, et al. Barriers, challenges and way forward for implementation of person-centered care model of patient and physician consultation: A survey of patients' perspective from eastern Mediterranean countries. Middle East Journal of Family Medicine. 2015;13(3):4-11

[8] Qidwai W, Khoja Tawfik AM, Salman R, Alnaser Faisal A, et al. Primary health care in pandemics: Barriers, challenges, and opportunities. World Family Medicine. 2021;19(8):6-11

[9] WHO. Seventy Countries Convene to Step Up Primary Health Care. Available from: https://www.who.int/news/item/23-10-2023-seventy-countries-convene-to-step-up-primary-health-care

[10] Rouleau K, Bourget M, Chege P, et al. Strengthening primary care through family medicine around the world: Collaborating toward promising practices. Family Medicine. 2018;50(6):426-436. DOI: 10.22454/FamMed.2018.210965

[11] Alnasir FA, Jaradat AA-K. The effect of training in primary health care centers on medical students' clinical skills. ISRN Family Medicine. 18 Apr 2013:403181. DOI: 10.5402/2013/403181

[12] McWhinney I. Family medicine in perspective. The New England Journal of Medicine. 1975;293:176-181

[13] Kidd M. The Contribution of Family Medicine to Improving Health Systems: A Guidebook from the World Organization of Family Doctors. 2nd ed. London: Radcliffe; 2013

[14] Alnaser FA. Role of family doctors and primary health care in COVID-19 pandemic. World Family Medicine/Middle East Journal of Family Medicine. 2020;18(9):61-66. DOI: 10.5742MEWFM.2020.93857

[15] Qidwai W, Nanji K, Khoja TAM, Rawaf S, AlKurashi NY, Alnasir F, et al. Health promotion, disease prevention, and periodic health checks: Perceptions

and practice among family physicians in Eastern Mediterranean region. Middle East Journal of Family Medicine. 2015;**13**(5):44-51

[16] Rawaf S, Qidwai W, Khoja TAM, Nanji K, Kurashi NY, Alnasir F, et al. New leadership model for family physicians in the Eastern Mediterranean region: A pilot study across selected countries. Journal of Family Medicine. 2017;**4**(2):1-7

[17] Alshammari SA. Preparedness to implement "a family physician for every family," which is the magic recipe for cost-effective health Care for all: Viewpoint. Journal of Nature and Science of Medicine. 2023;**6**(2):95-100

[18] Gutierrez C, Scheid P. The History of Family Medicine and Its Impact in US Health Care Delivery. Available from: https://www.aafpfoundation. org/content/dam/foundation/ documents/who-we-are/cfhm/ FMImpactGutierrezScheid.pdf

[19] Freeman TR. The Origins of Family Medicine, McWhinney's Textbook of Family Medicine. 4th ed. New York: Oxford Academic; 2016; online edn, Available from: https://academic.oup. com/book/24562/chapter-abstract/18780 6988?login=false&redirected From=

[20] Torell E. UNMC History: Family Medicine Pioneers. Available from: https:// www.unmc.edu/newsroom/2023/10/10/ unmc-history-family-medicine-pioneers/

[21] Faisal A. Abu baker Mohd Alrazi his input and achievements. Medical Arabization, The Journal of the Arabization Centre for Medical Sciences. 2010;**30**:42-44

[22] Faisal A. Physician characteristics across Medevils. Medical Arabization, The Journal of the Arabization Centre for Medical Sciences. 2009;**25**:95-101

[23] Brazier Y. Why Was Medieval Islamic Medicine Important? 2018. Available from: https://www.medicalnewstoday. com/articles/323612

[24] Mohamed K, Al-Ghazal SK. The significant influence and contributions of Al-Razi (Rhazes) to the establishment of pharmacy during the middle ages. Journal of the British Islamic Medical Association. 2020;**3**:1-4. Available from: https://www.jbima.com/article/the-significant-influence-and-contributions-of-al-razi-rhazes-to-the-establishment-of-pharmacy-during-the-middle-ages/

[25] A-Razi. Available from: https:// science4fun.info/al-razi/

[26] Tibi S. Al-Razi and Islamic medicine in the 9th century. Journal of the Royal Society of Medicine. 2006;**99**(4):206-207. Available from: https://www.ncbi.nlm. nih.gov/pmc/articles/PMC1420785/

[27] Abu Bakr al-Razi. How Early Islamic Science Advanced Medicine. 28-Víctor Pallejà de Bustinza. Available from: https://en.wikipedia.org/wiki/Abu_Bakr_ al-Razi; https://www.nationalgeographic. com/history/history-magazine/article/ muslim-medicine-scientific-discovery-islam

[28] Martyn Shuttleworth. Islamic Medicine. Available from: https:// explorable.com/islamic-medicine

[29] Medicine in the medieval Islamic world. Available from: https:// en.wikipedia.org/wiki/Medicine in_the_medieval_Islamic_world

[30] Yvette Brazier. Why Was Medieval Islamic Medicine Important? 2018. Available from: https://www. medicalnewstoday.com/articles/323612

[31] Lindberg DC, Shank MH. Medicine In Medieval Islam. Cambridge

University Press; 2013. Available from: https://www.cambridge.org/core/ books/abs/cambridge-history-of-science/medicine-in-medieval-islam/ B5CED270387C3D73CAF4439CD8716E31

[32] Katz B. A Medieval Arabic Medical Text Was Translated into Irish, Discovery Shows Ibn Sīnā's Canon of Medicine; 2019. Available from: https://www.smithsonianmag.com/ smart-news/medieval-arabic-medical-text-was-translated-irish-discovery-shows-180971669/

[33] Pormann P, Savage-Smith E. Medieval Islamic Medicine (the New Edinburgh Islamic Surveys). 1st ed. Edinburgh University Press; 2007. Available from: https://www.amazon.com/Medieval-Islamic-Medicine-PORMANN/ dp/0748620672

[34] Ali S. Medical education in medieval Islam. Hektoen International. 2013;5(3). Available from: https://hekint.org/2017/01/29/ medical-education-in-medieval-islam/

[35] Alvarez MC. The case history in medieval Islamic medical literature: Tajārib and Mujarrabāt as source. Medical History. 2010;54(2):195-214. Available from: https://www.ncbi.nlm. nih.gov/pmc/articles/PMC2844281/

[36] Amru Aginta Sebayang. Primary Health Care, The History, and Its Importance. 2023. Available from: https:// cisdi.org/en/article/primary-health-care-the-history-and-its-importance

[37] Rifkin SB. Alma Ata after 40 years: Primary health care and health for all-from consensus to complexity. BMJ Global Health. 2018;3(Suppl 3):e001188

[38] Declaration of Alma-Ata. Available from: https://en.wikipedia.org/wiki/ Declaration_of_Alma-Ata

[39] Declaration of ALMA-ATA. International Conference on Primary Health Care, Alma-Ata, USSR, 6-12 September 1978. Available from: https:// www3.paho.org/english/dd/pin/alma-ata_declaration.htm

[40] World Health Organization. World Health Organization Primary Health Care: Report of the International Conference on Primary Health Care Alma Ata, USSR, 6-12 September 1978. Geneva, Switzerland: World Health Organization; 1978

[41] Alma Ata Primary Healthcare Conference. Report of the Conference on Primary Healthcare, Alma Ata. Available from: https:// www.unicef.org/documents/ alma-ata-primary-healthcare-conference

[42] Alma-Ata Declaration. Available from: https://www. safeopedia.com/ definition/5337/alma-ata-declaration

[43] World Health Organization. Ottawa Charter for Health Promotion. World Health Organization; 1986. Available from: http://www.who.int/ healthpromotion/conferences/previous/ ottawa/en/

[44] WHO. Primary Health Care - Now more than Ever. WHO; 2008. Available from: https://www.who.int/director-general/speeches/detail/primary-health-care---now-more-than-ever

[45] Freeman J. Family medicine across the globe: Developing effective solutions. Family Medicine. 2018;50(6):417-419

[46] WHO. Report of the Global Conference on Primary Health Care: From Alma-Ata Towards Universal Health Coverage and the Sustainable Development Goals. Available from: https://www.who.int/ publications-detail-redirect/

[47] Declaration of Astana. 2018. Available from: https://www.who. int/publications-detail-redirect/ WHO-HIS-SDS-2018.61

[48] Declaration on Primary Health Care: Astana. 2018. Available from: https://www.rets.epsjv.fiocruz.br/en/ news/declaration-primary-health-care-astana-2018

[49] Willard WR, Land RL, Longmire WP, Williams CH, Johnson AJ, Michaelson J, et al. Meeting the Challenge of Family Practice. Chicago, IL: AMA; 1966

[50] Lee Burnett, DO. Unintended Consequences of 1960s Health Care Reform. Available from: https:// coastalresearch.org/2020/05/16/ unintended-consequences-of-1960s-health-care-reform/

[51] Schwartz CC, Ajjarapu AS, Stamy CD, Schwinn DA. Comprehensive history of 3-year and accelerated US medical school programs: A century in review. Medical Education Online. 2018;23(1):1530557

[52] Dalen JE, Ryan KJ, Alpert JS. Where have the generalists gone? They became specialists, then subspecialists. The American Journal of Medicine. 2017;130(7):766-768

[53] Taylor RB. The promise of family medicine: History, leadership, and the age of Aquarius. The Journal of the American Board of Family Medicine. 2006;19(2):183-190

[54] Family Medicine Scientific Council. Available from: https://www.arab-board. org/Specialties/Family-Medicine

[55] Faisal A. Family medicine in the Arab world? Is it a luxury? Journal of the Bahrain Medical Society. 2009;21(1):191-192

[56] Middle East Region Overview. Exploring Global Family Medicine - Wilfrid Laurier University; 2019. Available from: https:// globalfamilymedicine.org/ regionoverview-57

[57] Arya N, Gibson C, Ponka D, Haq C, Hansel S, Dahlman B, et al. Family medicine around the world: Overview by region: The Besrour papers: A series on the state of family medicine in the world. Canadian Family Physician. 2017;63(6):436-441. Available from: https://www.ncbi.nlm.nih.gov/pmc/ articles/PMC5471080/

[58] Qidwai W, Ashfaq T, Khoja TAM, Merchant K, Seneviratne A, Fahim AE, et al. equity in healthcare: Status, barriers, and challenges. Middle East Journal of Family Medicine. 2011;9(6):36-41

[59] Stewart M, Ryan B. Ecology of health care in Canada. Canadian Family Physician. 2015;61:449-453, (Eng), e249-54

[60] Kolber MR, Korownyk CS, Young J, Garrison S, Kirkwood J, Allan GM. The value of family medicine: An impossible job, done impossibly well. Canadian Family Physician. 2023;69(4):269-270

[61] Shi L. The relationship between primary care and life chances. Journal of Health Care for the Poor and Underserved. 1992;3:321-335

[62] Shi L, Macinko J, Starfield B, Wulu J, Regan J, Politzer R. The relationship between primary care, income inequality, and mortality in the United States, 1980-1995. Journal of the American Board of Family Practice. 2003;16:412-422

[63] Macinko J, Starfield B, Shi L. Quantifying the health benefits of

primary care physician supply in the United States. International Journal of Health Services. 2007;**37**(1):111-126

[64] Gulliford MC. Availability of primary care doctors and population health in England: Is there an association? Journal of Public Health Medicine. 2002;**24**:252-254

[65] Starfield B, Shi L, Macinko J. Contribution of primary care to health systems and health. The Milbank Quarterly. 2005;**83**(3):457-502. DOI: 10.1111/j.1468-0009.2005.00409.x

[66] Gulliford MC, Jack RH, Adams G, Ukoumunne OC. Availability and structure of primary medical care services and population health and health care indicators in England. BMC Health Services Research. 2004;**4**:12

[67] Pantoja T, Barreto J, Panisset U. Improving public health and health systems through evidence informed policy in the Americas. BMJ. 2018;**362**:k2469. Available from: https://www.bmj.com/content/362/bmj.k2469

[68] MacDonald T, Green L. A Cluster Analysis Exploring the Relationship between Daily Patient Volume, Provider Panel Size, Service Day Provision and Patient Health Outcomes in Alberta General Practitioner Practices. Oral Presentation in Family Medicine Summit March 6, 2020

[69] If There's a Doctor in the Family, Health Outcomes Improve. NBER. Available from: https://www.nber.org/digest/jun19/if-theres-doctor-family-health-outcomes-improve

[70] Pavlic DR, Sever M, Klemenc-Ketis Z, et al. Process quality indicators in family medicine: Results of an international comparison.

BMC Family Practice. 2015;**16**:172. Available from: https://bmcprimcare.biomedcentral.com/articles/10.1186/s12875-015-0386-7

[71] Bağcı H, Egici MT, Öztaş D, Gençer MZ, Mercan GN. The effect of family medicine implementation on primary health care services: Northeast Anatolia region evaluation. Haydarpasa Numune Medical Journal. 2021;**61**(2):209-216

[72] Sans-Corrales M, Pujol-Ribera E, Gené-Badia J, Pasarín-Rua MI, Iglesias-Pérez B, Casajuana-Brunet J. Family medicine attributes related to satisfaction, health and costs. Family Practice. 2006;**23**(3):308-316

[73] 4 Perks of Being a Family Physician SGU School of Medicine. Available from: https://www.sgu.edu/blog/medical/perks-of-becoming-a-family-physician/

[74] The Advantages of Having a Family Doctor. Available from: https://www.signaturefamilyhealth.com/blog/the-advantages-of-having-a-family-doctor

[75] Knight JC, Mathews M, Aubrey-Bassler K. Relation between family physician retention and avoidable hospital admission in Newfoundland and Labrador: A population-based cross-sectional study. CMAJ Open. 2017;**5**(4):E746-E752

[76] Rebolho RC, Poli Neto P, Pedebôs LA, Garcia LP, Vidor AC. Do family doctors refer less? Impact of FCM training on the rate of PHC referrals. Ciência & Saúde Coletiva. 2021;**26**(4):1265-1274. Portuguese, English

[77] O'Cathain A, Brazier JE, Milner PC, Fall M. Cost effectiveness of minor surgery in general practice: A prospective comparison with hospital practice. The

British Journal of General Practice. 1992;**42**(354):13-17

[78] Nelligan I, Montacute T, Browne MA, Lin S. Impact of a family medicine minor procedure service on cost of Care for a Health Plan. Family Medicine. 2020;**52**(6):417-421

[79] Liddy C, Drosinis P, Armstrong CD, McKellips F, Afkham A, Keely E. What are the cost savings associated with providing access to specialist care through the Champlain BASE eConsult service? A costing evaluation. BMJ Open Access. 2016;**6**(6):e010920

[80] Khanna N. Primary care cost savings—The role of trust. Family Practice. 2019;**36**(5):531-532, Available from: https://academic.oup.com/fampra/article/36/5/531/5373130?login=false

[81] 5 Benefits of Family Medicine Nation's Best Family Health Care. Available from: https://nationsbesthealth.com/5-benefits-of-family-medicine/

[82] Hellenberg D, Williams FR, Kubendra M, Kaimal RS. Strengths and limitations of a family physician. Journal of Family Medicine and Primary Care. 2018;**7**(2):284-287

[83] Ohta R, Ueno A, Kitayuguchi J, Moriwaki Y, Otani J, Sano C. Comprehensive care through family medicine: Improving the sustainability of aging societies. Geriatrics (Basel). 2021;**6**(2):59. Available from: https://www.ncbi.nlm.nih.gov/pmc/articles/PMC8293036/

[34] Mohammadibakhsh R, Aryankhesal A, Sohrabi R, Alihosseini S, Behzadifar M. Implementation challenges of family physician program: A systematic review on global evidence. Medical Journal of the Islamic Republic

of Iran. 2023;**37**:21. Available from: https://www.ncbi.nlm.nih.gov/pmc/articles/PMC10167646/

[85] de Almeida PF, Ligia G, Schenkman S, et al. Perspectives for primary health care public policy in South America. Ciênc. Saúde Coletiva. 2024;**29**(7):e03792024

[86] Stevens RA. The Americanization of family medicine: Contradictions, challenges, and change, 1969-2000. Family Medicine. 2001;**33**:232-243. Available from: https://www.researchgate.net/publication/12012708_The_Americanization_of_Family_Medicine_Contradictions_Challenges_and_Change_1969-2000

[87] Von Pressentin KB, Mash BJ, Esterhuizen TM. Examining the influence of family physician supply on district health system performance in South Africa: An ecological analysis of key health indicators. African Journal of Primary Health & Family Medicine. 2017;**9**(1):e1-e10

[88] Mash R, Almeida M, Wong WCW, Kumar R, von Pressentin KB. The roles and training of primary care doctors: China, India, Brazil and South Africa. Human Resources for Health. 2015;**13**(1):93

[89] Qidwai W, Nanji K, Khoja TAM, Rawaf S, Al Kurashi NY, Alnasir F, et al. Are we ready for a person-centered care model for patient-physician consultation? A survey from family physicians and their patients of the East Mediterranean region. European Journal of Person-Centered Medicine. 2013;**1**:2

Chapter 3

Critical Discourse Analysis of the UK General Practice Patient Survey: An Insight into the Crisis in General Practice

Jennifer Chiok Foong Loke, Kah Wai Lee and Elizabeth Anne Lee

Abstract

General practice in the United Kingdom (UK) is not only the cornerstone of the National Health Services (NHS) but also an important building block of the NHS long-term plan. Providing free medical and public health services to all UK residents, general practice often acts as the most common entry point to the NHS. Consequently, patient experience in general practice is regularly assessed, and this is primarily through the General Practice Patient Survey (GPPS). The results of the GPPS play a key role in shaping the direction of the NHS as well as determining the survival of general practice. The general practice crisis as indicated by the GPPS along with other evaluative tools has influenced the establishment of primary care networks, to which the majority of funding has since been redirected away from individual GP service providers. Whilst the GPPS continued assessing patient experience to guide NHS strategies and determine the survival of general practice, worsening of the crisis in general practice was reported. Using Fairclough's critical discourse analysis, we aim to uncover the relationship between the GPPS and patient experience. The analysis was conducted in an attempt to offer plausible explanations of the worsening general practice crisis in the UK.

Keywords: critical discourse analysis, general practice, GP crisis, GP patient survey, primary care network

1. Introduction

In the United Kingdom (UK), primary and specialist healthcare, including family medicine and public health services, are provided free of charge to all UK residents through the National Health Service (NHS). General practice (GP), the main provider of family medicine within primary care, serves as the most common entry point for patients into the NHS. As a result, GP is not only the cornerstone of the NHS but also an important building block of the NHS long-term plan. Given its pivotal role in healthcare delivery, GP services are continually evaluated to ensure effectiveness.

IntechOpen

The General Practice Patient Survey (GPPS) was commissioned by the National Health Service England (NHSE) to Ipsos for establishing patient experiences in GP. Since its first administration in 2007 [1], the GPPS has always been used by NHSE to complement other data sources for planning primary care services and informing direction of the NHS. Hence, medical doctors as general practitioners, who are commonly referred to as '*GPs*' by the UK public, were not only encouraged but were also, at one point in 2009, incentivised to promote the use of the GPPS to obtain patient feedback [2]. Health researchers [3, 4] who saw values of the GPPS had also relied on the patient survey as a tool for understanding various health outcomes in healthcare services. Whilst the GPPS was heavily used to inform the direction of health services, the Care Quality Commission (CQC) as an independent regulator of GP has also used it to rate GP services, so much so that the GPPS not only influences the direction of primary healthcare delivery but also has an indirect control over the survival and existence of each NHS GP service provider.

In recent times between 2021 and 2023, the GPPS as an important tool to inform local health services delivery had indicated an all-time-high patient dissatisfaction [5, 6]. The result trends implied increasing workload challenges and intensifying workforce crisis, both of which contributed to problematic patient access [6, 7]. The problems encountered had grown exponentially that it is now widely known that general practice in the UK is in crisis [5–7]. The well-discussed GP crisis stems from a decline in the number of general practitioners through recruitment, retention and retirement issues [8]. The Additional Role Reimbursement Scheme (ARRS) was then introduced through primary care networks (PCNs) as a solution to address the reduced number of '*GPs*' [9]. This strategy had then led to redundancies and increased unemployment of '*GPs*' who did locum work [10], further reducing '*GPs*' numbers to fulfill high demands for appointments. Evidently, PCNs, the blueprint as a saving grace for GP services, had inadvertently led to increased public dissatisfaction with their GP services, and patient satisfaction rate hit a record low, worsening the GP crisis [6].

It is important to note that the ARRS based on PCN establishment in 2019 was guided by results of the GPPS, aimed at resolving the GP crisis with a focus to address problematic patient access to GP. To be specific, the PCN was conceived based on NHS promises to achieve proactive, personalised, well-coordinated and integrated care, so that demand for '*GP*' appointments can be reduced. It is critical to appreciate the ARRS was introduced on the promise for equitable primary healthcare. This resulted in additional funding being directed to support the ARRS, where many more non-medical healthcare professionals were employed through PCNs, in the belief that patient appointments in GP could be increased [7]. The persistent trend in reduced ratings of patient experience of GP and worsening GP crisis was therefore not expected.

Whilst the NHS pinned high hopes on PCNs, the increased concerted efforts and large investment to improve patient experience of GP had inversely resulted in a higher patient dissatisfaction rate in GP services. This led to the publishing of the 2024 version of the GPPS [11]. This new version of the GPPS was redeveloped with an intent for it to continue reflecting the way services by GP were delivered and how patients experienced them. The latest results based on this version fetched a better result with 3% improvement for overall experience (74% in 2024; 71% in 2023) [12, 13]. The modest improvement does not justify the high level of investments, more so when the observed improvement in the 2024 survey was associated with a 1.3% reduction of the national response rate from 28.6% in 2023 to 27.3% in 2024 [12, 13].

Whilst we made these comparisons, Williams et al. [1] had advised against doing so because of their concerns that the 2024 version of the GPPS included changes that were set out in the delivery plan for recovering access to primary care. The authors [1] had particularly warned about the absence of the elements of improved access based on technologies in all previous versions and advised that the results of the 2024 GPPS were the start of the new time series for the GPPS.

We acknowledged the advice by Williams et al. [1]. The comparisons were, in fact, made in light of our appreciation of the differences between the 2023's version and the latest version published in 2024. It is important to note that any contributing factors to today's GP crisis were multi-faceted, and any influences by the GPPS on participant responses cannot be taken lightly. In this regard, we suspect that the context(s) in which patients responded to the GPPS could also have the capacity to influence patient responses. Hence, one cannot and should not take patient experience, as derived from the GPPS on face value. In our analysis, we attempted to explain the relationship between the GPPS and patient experience, and we did so in a micro-context of general practice as well as at macro-level in today's NHS. This was done with an attempt to provide some plausible explanations for the continuing poor GPPS ratings and, more importantly, the worsening of the GP crisis we witnessed in the UK.

2. UK general practice patient survey: Its reliability, validity and credibility

The GPPS was first administered 17 years ago in 2007 on an annual basis. Two years later, between April 2009 and March 2011, it was frequently administered on a quarterly basis and, thereafter, reduced to a biannual basis between 2011 and 2016 before returning to an annual basis in 2017 [1]. Patients over 16 years of age were randomly selected, resulting in approximately 2.5 million out of the over 67 million UK population being invited to participate in the GPPS. Whichever format the GPPS was administered, continuing effort and investment were made year on year, to revise the GPPS for the survey to realistically reflect on GP service delivery and the way patients experienced it.

Despite investment of time and finances, the response rate of the GPPS hovered around 30%, and this fell lower since 2022. As 5% to 30% was generally considered an acceptable response rate for self-administered surveys to evaluate customer satisfaction [14], other than the regular reviews by Ipsos, the volume of research on the GPPS was small. Evidently, queries regarding its reliability, validity and credibility had only been raised in earlier days of the administration of the GPPS [15–17]. No recent studies were found to have challenged its validity and reliability. Certainly, no qualitative studies were conducted to review the influences of the GPPS on patient responses. Given the inability to achieve an excellent patient uptake, such that the GPPS continued to suffer a nonresponse bias of at least 70%, it is vital that we examine the GPPS through a critical lens. This is important, particularly when surveys have every potential to create participants' responses [18], yet conclusions drawn from a 30% response rate of a small and self-selected UK population were continuously used to guide NHS strategies and direction. In this chapter, we demonstrate the use of Fairclough's critical discourse analysis to make transparent the relationship between the UK GPPS and patient experience.

As we know, the regular review by Ipsos had resulted in many versions of the UK GPPS over the past 17 years. The 2024 version being the latest was a result of revision of the 2023 version. As the current study was concerned with the current worsening of the GP crisis, the 2023 [19] and 2024 [11] versions were used for the purpose of this analysis, and the focus would be on statements about the experience of GP. Prior to the analysis, we will proceed with discussing our choice of Fairclough's critical discourse analysis (CDA) for this study.

3. Fairclough's critical discourse analysis

CDA is a useful methodology to study the exertion of political, social and economic power relations through discursive events, so that a better understanding of their social implications can be achieved. Language is used not only to describe the things in question or events of interest but, more importantly, to explain the ways things were done and to make explicit the reasons by which the events were constructed [20].

Fairclough's approach to CDA is a three-dimensional framework for analysing the things and events, but all of these were in the form of text [21, 22]. A feature in his framework was his attempt to combine a theory of power based on Gramsci's hegemony with a theory of discourse practice based on the concept of interdiscursivity. Fairclough saw the connection between text and social practices as being mediated by discourse practice. The reason for a three-dimensional framework was that he believed that there were three inter-related processes of CDA, which were tied to three inter-related dimensions of discourse as follows:

1. The object of analysis (including verbal, visual, or verbal and visual texts);

2. The processes by means of which the object is produced and received (writing/speaking/designing and reading/listening/viewing) by human subjects; and

3. The socio-historical conditions which govern these processes (social order of discourse/genre).

Fairclough saw the three dimensions as distinct, but he considered each of these as inter-dependent entities. In view of this consideration, a dialectical approach to CDA was advocated for the following analyses:

1. Textual analysis (description);

2. Processing analysis (interpretation); and

3. Social analysis (explanation).

The use of Fairclough's CDA for this study was to guarantee the focus of textual analysis on the signifiers that made up the GPPS. In this way, the specific linguistic selections, the juxtapositioning, the sequencing and the layout of the texts within the survey could be made transparent. Once the historical determination of these selections was recognised, the way in which the choices of linguistic selections that were linked to the conditions of the possibility of text production, text interpretation and consumption could then be identified and, ultimately, appreciated.

The reason for Fairclough's CDA for this study was also because we share Fairclough's [21] view about linguistic selection, that it has an impact on society in the formation and application of a specific theory, ideology, belief and strategy, which is ultimately used to gain authoritative power within politics, economics and society. This three-dimensional framework was to ensure that CDA maintained the capacity to place any social analysis into connection with the fine detail of a particular instance of social practices, in a way which is simultaneously oriented to textual detail, text production, distribution as well as interpretation and consumption, all of which were set within wider social and cultural contexts. In other words, Fairclough's [22] three-dimensional analytic framework could ensure CDA of each phase is linked to one another in discourse analysis, such that textual, interpretational and social levels were analysed as interrelated entities.

What made Fairclough's approach to CDA a useful tool for explaining the association between the GPPS and the GP crisis was the underpinning concept of Fairclough's [21, 23] approach to CDA; that it was guided by his belief that expressed in the language were the different sections and groups in society. Fairclough [19] believed that the idea of common sense was developed and put into the minds of common people through the tactful use of language in such a brilliant way by the elite class that the common people find it difficult to resist to such beliefs and ideologies as are sent their way from the dominant class. With regard to the GPPS, albeit it being administered by Ipsos, it was by the NHS who is the authority for health services, that the use of Fairclough's approach for the analysis potentially expose any such ideologies. The purpose of CDA in this study was mainly to highlight and understand the said belief systems and to know how they were expressed and communicated to the public in general, based on the GPPS.

In summary, as guided by Fairclough's CDA [21–23], the main aim of this analysis was to understand the construct of statements within the GPPS. This would allow an explanation of the phenomenon we experience in today's GP crisis. In essence, the embarking on Fairclough's three-dimensional framework to analyse the GPPS was with the aims to:

1. Highlight impression markers in the GPPS;

2. Identify main concerns of the GPPS; and

3. Relate possible social and cultural impacts implied in the GPPS.

4. Analysis, observations and discussions

We analysed the three elements at their various levels: micro (the GPPS text), meso (the relationship between the GPPS and the respondents in general practice) and macro (the social events within general practice). All three elements are subject to textual processing and social analyses in a dialectical fashion, as illustrated in **Figure 1**.

4.1 Textual analysis

Textual analysis was first conducted and aimed at exploring the elements of cohesion, semantics and morphology within the GPPS. The analysis revealed that all versions of the GPPS are entitled 'GP Patient Survey'. Whilst it is clear that it is a general practice patient survey, the general public take '*GP*' to mean their

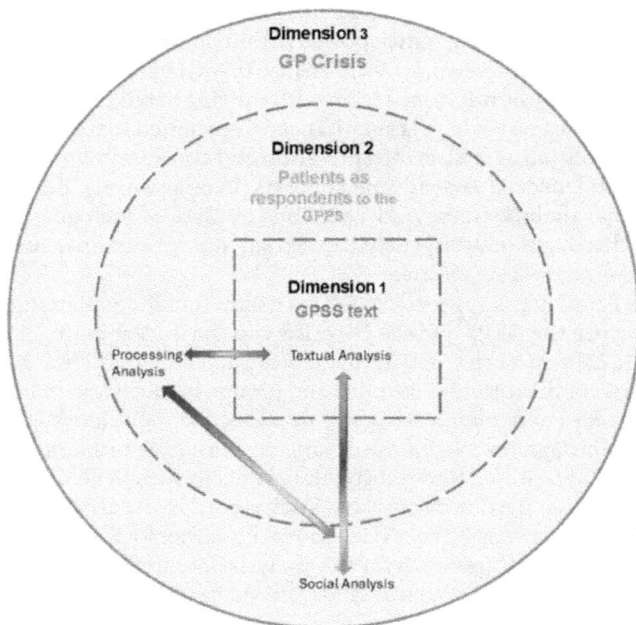

Figure 1.
Using Fairclough critical discourse analysis on the UK GPPS.

accountable medical doctor(s) who are the general practitioners, that the GPPS gave the impression that the purpose of the survey was to gather patients' view on their accountable medical doctor(s) and their services. Such impression of the GPPS continued into the title of the first section. 'Your local GP services' in the 2023 version [19] was even changed to 'Your GP practice services' in the 2024 version [11] to enhance the impression (**Figure 2**). Individuals who lack the contextual knowledge of the UK population would have mistakenly thought that the new heading comprised a typo as the amended version would read: 'Your General Practice Practice Services'. At this point, it is important that we reiterate the tacit knowledge of the UK population. In the UK, '*GP*' was a common abbreviation used by the public to mean their accountable family doctor, the general practitioner(s). By revising the first section of the 2024 version, to 'Your GP practice services', it reinforced the purpose of the survey as set in the title of the GPPS, that it was targeted at respondents who were registered

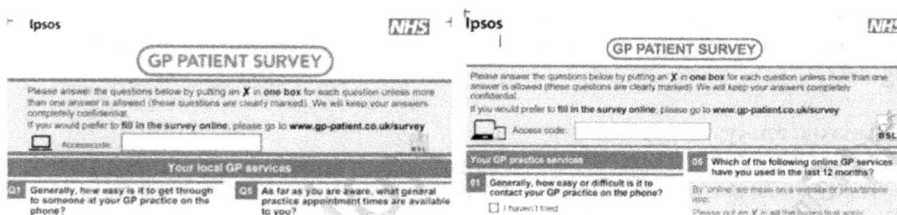

Figure 2.
UK GP Patient Surveys – 2023 and 2024 versions. GP Survey 2023 ([19], P. 1).

patients of their general practitioner's practice, to cast opinions of their accountable doctors and the services they provided.

Certainly, the section entitled 'Your GP practice services' was not a typo, but in fact a carefully crafted change in an attempt to ensure opinions of individual providers of general practice were gathered from the respondents. Whilst there was a strong desire to achieve answers from respondents about their own '*GP*', this was not clarified in the subsequent sections. In an attempt to achieve relevance of the GPPS, a new section on 'Pharmacy' was introduced in version 2024 [11] to reflect the current NHS context, where pharmacy services were encouraged at the PCN level through an 'integrated neighbourhood team'. However, the word 'Pharmacy' would instill the impression that an individual '*GP*' practice was the point of contact for any pharmaceutical matters. This was the case even if the pharmacy was an external organisation to the individual '*GP*' practice, which the respondent was registered with. Hence, this new section added confusions that was already introduced by the title of the survey and reinforced by the subtitle of first section. When information about patient experience on GP as a whole was required, as influenced by these titles, respondents were likely to attribute their accountable '*GPs*' for the services they received from the pharmacies, even when these were not part of the services offered by the general practitioners.

Similar confusion regarding pharmacies' service was found in the 2024's version in the section on 'Dentistry' [11]. The word 'NHS' no longer appeared before the word 'Dentistry' like it did in the 2023 version [19]. Obviously, this version was less clear about NHS being the context of dental services; nevertheless, the lack of the much-needed contextualised information was repaired in the individual statements for experience of dentistry, making it clearer to the respondents that the GPPS was eliciting patients' view on the NHS dentistry services. Given the shortage of NHS dental services in the UK – many of which have been privatised and, hence, costly – the frustration of being unable to access free dental care further contributed to patients' dissatisfaction. As a result, albeit putting statements about dental services in a separate section to reinforce awareness of the respondents that they were to focus on dental services in this section, the frustration respondents experienced in dental services would possibly have an influence on their ratings in all other sections of the GPPS.

Evidence of Ipsos's effort towards relevance was also seen in the changing of the subtitle in the second section to 'your last contact' in the 2024 version [11], rather than limiting it to 'making appointment' as seen in the 2023 version [19]. This change was also to reflect the reality of the current GP context when patients could contact their GP practice for a whole host of things other than making appointments. Respondents who saw the GP as a place to secure a doctor's appointment were also made aware of the various services which the GP surgery could be contacted for. Further effort to achieve relevance was seen in replacing the section of 'COVID-19' in version 2023 [19] with a statement to explore long COVID in version 2024 [11]. The revision reflected the acknowledgement of the possible change in individuals' health post-pandemic.

Other than the title and subtitles, both surveys comprised brief and straightforward statements in each section, with clear instructions to guide respondents. The lexical choices in the two GPPS appeared simple with only one aim, that was to obtain information about the individuals, their self-caring behaviours and their experiences. The discourse is clearly an institutional or, otherwise, an evaluative-type discourse to gather feedback, assess quality and make evaluations based on specific criteria. The response options lexicon indicated the aim for quality data. A wide range of options, which included neutral and negative options, were used to encourage thoughtful responses, aimed at capturing the full range of opinions and, at the same time, avoiding bias.

Statements in the GPPS were generally presented in two forms of text with two different intents as described by Bull et al. [24]; they were either 'patient reported experience measures' (PREMs) to capture 'what' and 'how' things happened during an encounter in GP or as 'patient reported outcome measures' (PROMs) to capture patients' subjective satisfaction measures of their GP encounters. Continued analysis of sections 1 to 4 in both GPPS revealed that the 2023 version has 15 PREMs and 17 PROMs and the 2024 version has 17 PREMs and 15 PROMs. It appeared that there was a good balance of PREMs and PROMs in the two GPPS; however, a close examination demonstrated that statements which took the form of PREMS were almost always linked to PROMs, and phrases such as 'Very easy', 'Not at all easy', 'Very helpful', 'Not at all helpful', 'Very satisfied' and 'Very dissatisfied' were often used. This strongly suggested the promotion of user-centredness, with an attempt to fulfil the ethos of the NHS constitution that 'The patient will be at the heart of everything the NHS does' [25]. However, the heavy employing of PROMs had directed focus of the responses to past encounter experiences. As such, PREMs which promoted the idea of healthcare quality as defined by the concepts of patient-centred, effective, efficient timely and equitable were less emphasised in both versions of the GPPS.

The attempt to emphasise subjective individual opinions was made explicit based on further textual analysis. Together the two sections of 'Your local GP services' and 'Making appointments' made up the highest number of 21 statements in the 2023 version [19]. Similarly, a high number of statements were found in 'Your GP practice services' (7 statements) and 'Your last contact' (9 statements) within the 2024 version [11]. The statements in the two sections suggested that the emphasis of the GPPS, might have been to reinforce NHS ethos of patient centredness, but the focus was more on administrative issues rather than doctor–patient relationship. The administrative emphasis was strengthened by the conditional and contextual lexical choices within the GPPS, all of which were tailored to the individual respondents, treating them as general consumers in an open market rather than patients. For example, statements were designed to explore how quick or how easy it was for patients to make contact with their GP (statements 1 to 3), whether GP staff on reception were helpful (statement 4), both of which could fetch positive ratings only if respondents felt that their requests were fulfilled. The lexical choices were then accompanied with a casual tone to impress the respondents that it was legitimate to take their position as consumers (in a general market) rather than as patients (within the NHS context). This concept was quite pronounced in statements 6 and 7, where the impression of prioritising patient choice for a specific healthcare professionals was established; so much so that the traditional concept of medical doctors' choices, as based on authoritative medical healthcare knowledge to provide care, were erased.

4.2 Processing analysis

Processing analysis was another stage of analysis we conducted. Although presented separately, this stage of analysis was conducted in conjunction with textual analysis and social analysis. For this stage, we focused on the way respondents were made to see themselves in these surveys, hence the focus on text generation, text interpretation and text consumption.

First and foremost, all UK residents are familiar with the discourse of '*GP* and patients', and being invitees to complete the GPPS, the position of patients in the UK who were entitled to free GP services by the NHS are reinforced in the GPPS. During the stage of textual analysis, we explained the meaning of '*GP*' in the perspective of the majority of the UK population, that the abbreviation was likely to mean the accountable general practitioners rather than the general practice, as intended by Ipsos. Presumably, the patient-medical doctor relationship was reinforced, simply by respondents having sight to the title 'GP patient survey'. Such a presumption would also account for patients' impression that the questions in the GPPS were related to their views on their '*GPs*', the individual accountable general practitioners and the services these medical doctors provided, as opposed to the GP services as a whole, as intended by the GPPS. In this regard, respondents were likely to hold individual '*GPs*' accountable for any experience they encountered in general practice.

Further processing analysis demonstrated the building of a customer–supplier relationship through the GPPS. Strong emphases on patient choices and the concerns about patient satisfaction were significant in both versions of the GPPS. The 2023 version had also opened up the respondents' mind, about their rights as 'customers' who were entitled to a wider range of choices. This was more significantly emphasised in the 2024 version. In the 2023 version, there were two statements in the first section and six in the second section about patient choices. However, the entire first and second sections of the 2024 version (statements 1 to 7; 9 to 10; 13 to 15) were devoted to emphasising patient choices, particularly with access to their '*GPs*' (statements 6, 7, 19, 20, 22). The various ways for securing GP appointments, including the NHS App, which was similar to online shopping, where respondents, as desired, could book appointments online and also, cancel it as and when they liked, without reason to their '*GP*' practice, was introduced. This newly introduced convenience unrealistically raised patient expectations about securing appointments with their '*GPs*'. When patients contacted their '*GP*' practice and expected an appointment with their accountable general practitioner, but were triaged to receive care from a non-medical professional based on the ARRS, they were likely to be more dissatisfied than before.

The GPPS also measures respondents' satisfaction by their subjective opinion, particularly regarding the speed of GP services. These were seen in three statements (11, 15, 20) in the 2023 version and seven statements (11, 12, 13, 15, 19–21) in the 2024 version. All these statements were then linked to a subjective satisfaction rating. It appeared that the criteria of GP services were benchmarked against customer services, those of which we experienced in fast food chains, Uber Taxi service or Amazon Prime. These are retail markets whereby services and products were supplied upon customers' demand where customers' convenience was the priority. The revised 2024 version had a stronger emphasis on '*GP's*' responsibility for speedy GP services to a greater extent than the 2023 version.

These changes in the 2024 version reinforced the asymmetric customer (patients)–supplier ('*GP*') relationship that was built in the 2023 version. Consequently, '*GPs*' are further pushed to focus on speed and 'customer choices' in their service delivery, whilst not expected to give up on quality and details as guided by professional practice and ethics. As the GPPS evolved, in the name to 'reflect' reality in GP, it is observed to have exerted a power to mould GP into a business, similar to those set within an open market, but without the same level of resources of a private business.

4.3 Social analysis

Social analysis is the continuing analysis from textual and process analyses to explain the social norm of GP. The focus on the macro-contexts of the GPPS leads us to a better understanding of the worsening of the UK GP crisis [7]. As early as year 2000, GP faced a continuing significant and growing strain. This phenomenon has worsened over the last decade and became such a serious concern in recent years, that lately, the UK GP crisis was frequently covered in the UK media and political discourse. There were concerns that the GP crisis could spiral out of control, and the concerns of rising patient demand and increasingly undervaluing of the work in GP [7] were raised in light of the results of the GPPS.

Amongst many problematic issues in GP, the lack of appointments has been identified as the crux of the GP crisis. As discussed earlier, this was due to the drop in volume of 'GPs' resulting from retirement as well as purposeful replacement of 'GPs' based on the ARRS. The crisis worsened because in the midst of diminishing GP numbers, there was increasing patients' felt need of urgent medical attention, which could only be delivered by a 'GP' and that it must be provided by the patients' preferred 'GP'. It is very common that patients who experienced a slight burning sensation on micturition, or a tickly cough, would call their GP practice on the first few days of these symptoms. Since 'advised' by the GPPS, that they could request a same-day appointment, and have a choice to the pool of healthcare professionals, these patients were likely to contact their 'GP' practice demanding to be seen urgently and would consider a satisfied encounter only after having been prescribed with 'something' by their preferred 'GPs'.

In many GP practices which deliver healthcare services responsibly, these patients were likely to be turned down by the staff at the front desk. They would not be given any appointments, let alone a 'GP' appointment. Instead, the necessary advice on self-caring behaviours will be offered; they might also be triaged to community pharmacists (non-medical professionals) for homely remedies. These care paths were in contrast to what patients had come to expect. The previous analyses demonstrated that respondents were led to believe they had the choice of their 'GPs' for pharmaceutical services. Consequently, even if the care was triaged appropriately to the pharmacies, patients would still contact their 'GP' practices for matters that should have been handled by these other non-'GP' organisations.

There were many other unnecessary contacts made to the 'GP' practice, which compounded the GP crisis. One very common example was patient contacts about referrals that were made to specialist care. Despite patients being repeatedly advised that their care needs were triaged and placed on a waiting list, patients would still contact their 'GP' practice, requesting their referrals to secondary care to be expedited or, otherwise, to have a conversation with their 'GPs' and demanded the reason from the 'GPs' for the (extended) delayed care by others. Other than this, frequent contacts also arose from patients having to rebook appointments after failing to attend those scheduled, very often due to patient's preference to prioritise an all-inclusive holiday or an appointment made with a plumber or an electrician over a GP appointment.

So far, our discussions of the GP crisis might have led to the belief that the problems were limited to the front desks; in reality, patient demand had become so intense that it often spilled over to the consultation rooms. During any consultations that were held in GP, gone were the days when patients provided the signs and symptoms to help facilitate a clinical decision by qualified healthcare professionals. More often than not, patients come to their 'GP' with long lists of self-perceived diagnoses, holding a strong but skewed view that 'patients know best' (as in customer knows what to purchase), to then justify their demand for an avalanche of medications and medical investigations such as bloods and imaging tests. In the name of patient empowerment and patient choice, and the desire for a good GPPS scores, there were increased pressure to practice defensive medicine. By meeting patient desires, GP staff at all levels became overwhelmed with a large amount of workload arose from the large volume of medical investigations and test results.

The above few examples were real case scenarios taken from a local context, which are commonly observed in other parts of the UK. Whilst there was increased patient demand, patient desires were not, and cannot, always be fulfilled by any staff in GP, including the patients' own '*GPs*'. It was evidenced that the patient wants could never be fulfilled in the same extent they would have, in an open retail market by the suppliers. Failing to have patient wants fulfilled by the '*GPs*', as defined by the GPPS, had then led to patient complaints, which further added to the overwhelming workload or, otherwise, verbal abuse from patients [26].

Our social analysis of the GP crisis demonstrated that the patient dominance, as achieved through the GPPS, has changed the rules of patient–GP relationships to have resulted in today's GP crisis. This observation was based on the assumption that successful completion of the GPPS required respondents' time and effort to go through the text within the GPPS, and more importantly, it required respondents to internalise the concepts within it [18]. Our analysis demonstrated that the GPPS was a typical hegemonic situation, where (NHS) dominance over GP is achieved through control of legitimating ideas (of the respondents) and norms (patient demands), thus ensuring the hegemon dictates the 'rules' of GP provision. All of these were, in fact, found in the General Medical Services (GMS) contracts [27] that tied '*GPs*' to a range of mandatory health and social services within a context of diminishing resources. Just to name a few, provision of online services, enhanced patient access to GP beyond the normal contractual hours, self-bookable appointments, same-day appointments or no more than 14-day appointments from patient contact and so on. The change in terms of the GMS contract in favour of the patients were then repeatedly instilled in patients through their responding of the GPPS where patient convenience and desires are legitimately prioritised over appropriateness of care based on illness and health.

5. Conclusions

Our analysis revealed a hegemonic approach in the GPPS, which shaped the patient-GP relationship. Clearly, embedded in the GPPS discourse was the promotional discourse set within a customer-GP practice discourse. Patients going through the statements of the GPPS were instilled with a strong belief in patient choice and the concept of just-in-time service, similar to or even better than what patients would experience in the open market. In this regard, the GPPS had acted as a tool for building an asymmetric patient–GP relationship in favour of the patients. Our analysis demonstrated that the GPPS provided the platform where this hegemonic relationship evolved from the imbalanced power of a patient over their '*GPs*'. At face value, the GPPS were sent to individuals on a yearly basis to ostensibly elicit patient feedback on the NHS services, in reality, it subliminally exerted the power of influence, to generate the common-sense normalcy of mundane practice as the basis of continuity and reproduction of power relations between the patients and their '*GPs*'. In essence, through its constant determinedly and unilaterally imposing dominance and power, the GPPS exerted influence over the patients, that it facilitated the positioning of hegemony at the meta-level which represented a spatial domain impacting the mental models of the respondents who then legitimised their social practices (continuing unreasonable demands on '*GPs*') and ideas (an impression about patient rights as 'customers') to legitimise their continuing unreasonable demands.

Our analysis demonstrated that the GPPS exemplifies a modern discourse, characterised by the distinctive important role in the constitution and reproduction of power-relations, specifically between patients and their '*GPs*'. It constructs social identities that transition patients into customers, altering their expectations of GP services. Our findings clarified that the GPPS is not merely a feedback tool for gathering patient experience of GP services, but it actively reshapes how respondents perceive GP services. As patient expectations diverge from what is realistically and ethically feasible, the crisis within the UK GP system is likely to escalate. On top of this, the continuing use of results as derived from a 30% response rate of a small and self-selected UK population to guide NHS strategies and direction, continue to risk resource misallocation, GP crisis exacerbation and ultimately public trust in GP. If these trends continue, we risk a future where general practice may cease to exist. To ensure the sustainability of GP services in the NHS, it is crucial to revise the GPPS. It should be transformed into an educational tool that enhances public understanding of healthcare realities. By grounding patients' perceptions in the practical context of general practice, we can foster a more equitable and productive patient-GP relationship, ultimately improving the overall UK health system.

Acknowledgements

We thank Mr. Bryant K Lee and Dr. Deborah K H Lim for reviewing the final drafts of our work.

Conflict of interest

The authors declare no conflict of interest.

Author details

Jennifer Chiok Foong Loke*, Kah Wai Lee and Elizabeth Anne Lee
Park View Surgery, Hessle, England

*Address all correspondence to: jennifer.loke@nhs.net; jennifercfloke@yahoo.com

IntechOpen

References

[1] Williams R, Gray M, Weigold E. GP Patient Survey: Questionnaire Redevelopment Report. London: Ipsos; 2023. Available from: https://www.gp-patient.co.uk/downloads/2024/qandletter/GPPS%202024%20Questionnaire_redevelopment_report_PUBLIC.pdf [Accessed: October 6, 2024]

[2] Farrington C, Burt J, Boiko O, Campbell J, Roland M. Doctors' engagements with patient experience surveys in primary and secondary care: A qualitative study. Health Expectations. 2016;3:385-394. DOI: 10.1111/hex.12465

[3] Carter M, Roland M, Cambell J, Brearley S. Using the GP Patient Survey: To Improve Patient Care: A Guide for General Practices. London: National Primary Care Research & Development Centre. Available from: https://www.gp-patient.co.uk/downloads/FINAL_GP_Handbook.pdf; 2009 [Accessed: September 28, 2024]

[4] Heald A, Stedman M, Lunt M, Livingston M, Cortes G, Gadsby R. General practice (GP) level analysis shows that patients' own perceptions of support within primary care as reported in the GP patient survey (GPPS) are as important as medication and services in improving glycaemic control. Primary Care Diabetes. 2020;4:29-32. DOI: 10.1016/j.pcd.2019.04.005

[5] O'Dowd A. GP patient survey: Getting an appointment is harder but decline in satisfaction slows. BMJ. 2023;382:1629. DOI: 10.1136/bmj.p1629

[6] Smail J. Public satisfaction with GP services hits record low. Nursing Practice. 2024;365. Available from: https://www.nursinginpractice.com/latest-news/public-satisfaction-with-gp-services-hits-record-low/ [Accessed: September 28, 2024]

[7] The Conversation Trust (UK) Limited. GP Crisis: How Did Things Go So Wrong, and What Needs to Change? UK: The Conversation Trust Limited; 2023. Available from: https://theconversation.com/gp-crisis-how-did-things-go-so-wrong-and-what-needs-to-change-208197 [Accessed: October 4, 2024]

[8] British Medical Association. Pressures in General Practice Data Analysis. United Kingdom: British Medical Association; 2024. Available from: https://www.bma.org.uk/advice-and-support/nhs-delivery-and-workforce/pressures/pressures-in-general-practice-data-analysis [Accessed: October 3, 2024]

[9] Loke JC, Lee KW. Additional roles reimbursement to primary care networks: An uplift or downfall of general practice partnership? British Journal of General Practice. 2023;74(738):38-39. DOI: 10.3399/bjgp24X736089

[10] The Guardian. Revealed: Locum GPs in England Can't Find Work as Surgeries Buckle under Patient Demand. United Kingdom: The Guardian. 2024. Available from: https://www.theguardian.com/society/article/2024/may/12/england-locum-gps-doctors-work-surgeries-british-medical-association; [Accessed: October 3, 2024]

[11] Ipsos. GP Survey 2024. United Kingdom: Ipsos; 2024. Available from: https://www.gp-patient.co.uk/downloads/2024/qandletter/GPPS%202024%20Questionnaire_PUBLIC.pdf [Accessed: October 6, 2024]

[12] Ipsos. 2024 GP Patient Survey Results Released. United Kingdom: Ipsos; 2024. Available from: https://www.ipsos.com/

en-uk/2024-gp-patient-survey-results-released [Accessed: September 28, 2024]

[13] Ipsos. 2023 GP Patient Survey Results Released. United Kingdom: Ipsos. Available from: https://www.ipsos.com/en-uk/2023-gp-patient-survey-results-released; 2023 [Accessed: September 28, 2024]

[14] Cleave P. What Is a Good Survey Response Rate? SmartSurvey. London. 2020. Available from: https://www.smartsurvey.co.uk/blog/what-is-a-good-survey-response-rate; [Accessed: September 28, 2024]

[15] Asprey A, Campbell JL, Newbould J, Cohn S, Carter M, Davey A. Challenges to the credibility of patient feedback in primary healthcare settings: A qualitative study. The British Journal of General Practice. 2013;**63**:e200-e2e8. DOI: 10.3399/bjgp13X664252

[16] Davey AF, Roberts MJ, Mounce L, Maramba I, Campbell JL. Test–retest stability of patient experience items derived from the national GP patient survey 2016. Springer Plus. 1755;5:1-15. DOI: 10.1186/s40064-016-3377-9

[17] Mounce LT, Barry HE, Calitri R, Henley WE, Campbell J, Roland M, et al. Establishing the validity of English GP patient survey items evaluating out-of-hours care. BMJ. 2016;**25**(11):842-850. DOI: 10.1136/bmjqs-2015-004215

[18] Tourangeau R, Rips LJ, Rasinski K. The Psychology of Survey Response. UK: Cambridge University Press; 2012. DOI: 10.1017/CBO9780511819322

[19] Ipsos. GP Survey 2023. United Kingdom: Ipsos. 2023. Available from: https://gp-patient.co.uk/downloads/2023/qandletter/GPPS_2023_Questionnaire_PUBLIC.pdf; [Accessed: September 28, 2024]

[20] Loke JC-F, Coluquhoun D, Lee K-W. Critical Discourse Analysis of Interprofessional Online Learning in Health Care Education. USA: Nova Science Publishers Inc.; 2011. ISBN: 9781611227291

[21] Fairclough N. Language and Power. London: Longman; 2001

[22] Fairclough N. Critical Discourse Analysis. London: Longman; 1995

[23] Fairclough N. Critical discourse analysis and marketization of public discourse. Discourse and Society. 1993;**4**(2):133-168. DOI: 10.1177/0957926593004002002

[24] Bull C, Byrnes J. A systematic review of the validity and reliability of patient-reported experience measures. Health Services Research. 2019;**54**:1023-1035. DOI: 10.1111/1475-6773.13187

[25] The NHS Constitution for England. [Department of Health and Social Care]. 2023. Available from: https://www.gov.uk/government/publications/the-nhs-constitution-for-england/the-nhs-constitution-for-england#:~:text=4.,it%20to%20improve%20its%20services

[26] Wilkinson E. Almost all General Practice Staff Have Been Verbally Abused, Study Finds. United Kingdom: PULSE. 2024. Available from: https://www.pulsetoday.co.uk/news/special-investigations/gp-abuse/almost-all-general-practice-staff-have-been-verbally-abused-study-finds/; [Accessed: October 4, 2024]

[27] NHS England. Standard General Medical Services Contract. England: NHS England; 2024. Available from: https://www.england.nhs.uk/wp-content/uploads/2024/08/PRN01358i-standard-general-medical-services-contract-august-2024-v2.pdf [Accessed: October 6, 2024]

Chapter 4

Maintenance of Cold Chain during Immunisation: Voices of Learner Nurses

Takalani Edith Mutshatshi and Thabo Arthur Phukubye

Abstract

Maintenance of cold chain is integral for vaccine potency maintenance. Most vaccines are temperature-sensitive, hence cold chain maintenance is essential. Cold chain is crucial to keep the potency of vaccines. Improper vaccine storage and handling affect the quality of administered vaccines as lost potency of vaccines cannot be replaced. Nurses must maintain cold chain to maintain their lifespan until administration to clients. Learner nurses at a public university in Limpopo province, South Africa share their experiences on cold chain maintenance during immunisation. The objectives were to explore and describe the maintenance of cold chains during immunisation in clinical areas as voiced by learner nurses. A qualitative, explorative, descriptive, and contextual research design was used. A non-probability purposive sampling method was used to select participants. Data was collected through a semi-structured interview, using an interview guide. Data was analysed using Tesch's open coding method. Measures were taken to ensure trustworthiness and that ethical issues were adhered to. The findings of the study revealed a shortage of resources and a lack of knowledge and skills. The study recommends the provision of adequate resources, involvement of nurses in determining training needs, in-service training, and provision of a backup system for power interruptions.

Keywords: learner nurse, voices, cold chain, maintenance, immunisation

1. Introduction

Maintenance of the vaccine cold chain is integral concerning transportation, storage, handling, and administering. Administration of vaccines is the way to control the spread of viruses however, vaccination programmes across the globe are faced with challenges that are associated with the vaccine cold chain management and cold storage facilities. Cold chain management is aimed at ensuring vaccine potency to effectively protect individuals against vaccine-preventable diseases [1]. Cold chain management is crucial in keeping the potency and stability of vaccines as vaccines are heat sensitive and some vaccines are also affected by freezing [2]. Effective maintenance of the cold chain is essential to ensure stability and potency of the vaccines as most vaccines are temperature-sensitive and prolonged exposure to temperatures outside the range of +2°C and + 8°C can impact vaccine potency. Furthermore, regular renewal of cold chain infrastructure, continuous staff training and monitoring of effective immunisation coverage were recommended approaches to improve the cold chain [1, 3]. Collectively, through an enabling global and in-country environment, cold chain problems which act as a substantial barrier to effective and full immunisation coverage can be eliminated [4].

The World Health Organisation (WHO) guidelines and manufacturer product inserts recommend that all vaccines except OPV be kept at 2–8°C. Immunisation as a preventive health effort to provide immunity to specific diseases has shown its effectiveness in reducing morbidity and mortality in children [5–7]. Once the potency of a vaccine is lost, it cannot be regained or restored, and the vaccine will no longer protect against the target disease [8]. A study conducted in Indonesia by [9] revealed that the application of cold chain in the storage of vaccines and delivery practices in 11 sub-district healthcare centres was not ideal, therefore requiring a need for improvement- through an intervention strategy.

A study conducted in Ethiopia shows that health professionals have limited knowledge of cold chain management, vaccine shake tests and different vaccines that are sensitive to heat, freeze and light [10]. The findings of a study conducted in Ghana recommend continuous professional education for cold chain, provision of adequate human, financial, and material resources for effective cold chain management, improved monitoring and evaluation of cold chain activities and supply the district with cold chain equipment and logistics [11, 12]. The constancy of the vaccine is highly determined by the availability of the required temperature, therefore good monitoring starting from the manufacturer up to the period of usage through maintenance of the cold chain is important [4, 5, 13].

Effective cold chain management systems are critical in conserving vaccines from production to vaccination sites. Some deficiencies in cold chain management include a lack of facilities and equipment conducive to cold chain management and a lack of knowledge and training on vaccine management by healthcare workers officers [14]. Refrigerators for vaccines have reportedly been found to be storing food, laboratory reagents and medicines in Lagos clinics [15]. There are still gaps in knowledge, skills, attitudes and a lack of adherence to cold chain management practices which impact the effective management of the cold chain system [16].

A study conducted in South Africa in Limpopo province by Mothiba and Tladi [17] revealed that the cold chain is not well-maintained during the transportation and storage of vaccines by the people who are supposed to take care of this process. Furthermore, nurses have the responsibility to maintain the cold chain and to ensure period and its lifespan must be maintained until it is administered to the patient and must be potent within the set period. Despite the significance of cold chain management in maintaining the potency of vaccines, gaps still exist in the capability of healthcare practitioners to maintain the cold chain effectively.

2. Clarifying key concepts

The key concepts used in this chapter are clarified below to enhance understanding.

2.1 Learner nurse

A learner nurse is a person undergoing education and training in nursing and must be registered with the South African Nursing Council (SANC) in accordance with the Nursing Act no 33 of 2005 as amended [18]. A learner nurse in this chapter is a student registered with the SANC to study a nursing programme at an accreditated Nursing Education Institution(NEI) of Limpopo province for a specified period. It is clear from the introduction that cold chain maintenance is a challenge to nurse practitioners worldwide and this impacts the effectiveness of administered vaccines.

2.2 Maintenance

Maintenance is promotive and preventive actions carried out to retain a system in an acceptable operating condition [19]. In this chapter, maintaining means keeping something in good condition and ensuring that all vaccines are kept at the desired temperature of 2–8 degrees Celsius and this is ensured until administered. From the introduction it was highlighted that some vaccines are temperature-sensitive and hence require strict measures to keep them at the correct temperatures.

2.3 Cold chain

According to the National Department of Health [3], cold chain refers to the system of the people, equipment, transport and procedures responsible for ensuring that vaccines reach the vaccine site having been maintained in the appropriate specified temperatures. In this chapter, a cold chain is a system used by nurses to keep the vaccines at the required temperatures of 2–8 degrees Celsius to ensure maximum effectiveness during immunisation. From the introduction, there are various challenges globally in the effective maintenance of cold chain due to a wide range of factors that need strategic intervention.

2.4 Voices

A voice is a muscular effort of the whole body in a purposeful way to release the sound in the form of an intended speech [20]. In this chapter, a voice is used as a metaphor indicating the concerns of nurses regarding the effects of the inadequate maintenance of the cold chain during immunisation and the importance of joining hands with other nurses towards improving cold chain maintenance.

2.5 Immunisation

Immunisation is a process where a suspension containing the dead or weakened organisms of a disease is injected into a person to immunise them against a specific disease [21, 22]. In this chapter, Immunisation is the method of giving an injection and or oral vaccine with a live or inactivated virus to an individual, child and or adult to prevent infectious diseases whereby the origin of infection and or the chain of the spread of disease is blocked thereby increasing the individual's resistance to that particular infection.

3. Research methods

3.1 Research approach

The study employed a qualitative approach to collect data from learner nurses on their views on cold chain maintenance. The qualitative research approach enabled the researcher to obtain rich and in-depth information on cold chain maintenance in healthcare institutions during immunisation.

3.2 Research design

The study adopted a qualitative, explorative, descriptive and contextual research design to explore and describe how cold chain is maintained during immunisation and this was done within the context, of the training environments which are healthcare facilities.

3.3 Population and sampling

The population comprised all registered learner nurses in their second, third and fourth years for the academic year and a total of 190 learner nurses. A non-probability purposive heterogeneous sampling method was used to select participants for the study following a predetermined inclusion criterion.

3.4 Data collection and analysis

Data was collected through semi-structured face-to-face interviews, using an interview guide. Data was collected until data saturation was achieved at Participant 17. Data was recorded using a voice recorder with the permission of participants and field notes were taken to capture the non-verbal cues. The interviews lasted for 30–45 minutes The collected data was transcribed verbatim along with the field notes. Data was analysed using Tesch's open coding method with the involvement of an independent coder where an agreement was reached in the development of themes and sub-themes.

4. Results

The data analysis yielded the following theme and sub-themes illustrated in **Table 1** below.

4.1 Shortage of resources

The study findings revealed that there is a shortage of resources. The following sub-themes were identified, shortage of staff, inadequate equipment and supplies and power supply interruptions.

4.1.1 Shortage of staff

This study indicates that there is a shortage of nurses responsible for immunisation in the clinic which affects cold chain maintenance negatively. It occurs when there is more workload than the number of health workers. The shortage of staff has been explained by Participant 1 who stated '*If the staff is not enough and there are lot of patients, the nurse working with immunisation will be under pressure and the cooler box will be opened and closed frequently and cold air will be lost*'.

Participant 3 said '*You find that nurses are attending to many patients and they end up not following protocols of maintaining cold chain because they can take out a vaccine and*

Theme	Sub-theme
4.1. Shortage of resources	4.1.1 Shortage of staff
	4.1.2 Inadequate equipment and supplies
	4.1.3. Power supply interruptions
4.2. Lack of knowledge and skills	4.2.1 Inadequate knowledge of cold chain maintenance
	4.2.2 Lack of in-service training on cold chain management
	4.2.3 Ignorance and negligence to adhere to cold chain principles
4.3. Suggestions to improve maintenance of cold chain	4.3.1 Provision of adequate equipment for cold chain management
	4.3.2 In-service training for nurses on cold chain management
	4.3.3 Provision of backup system for power interruptions

Table 1.
Themes and sub-themes.

put it out in the open and they will just be withdrawing vaccine without putting it back in the cooler box'.

Participant 4 *'With the cooler box...so many patients...so many kids to immunise...we sometimes lack time to go and check the cooler box to replace the icepacks....and those are the challenges that I experience'.*

The findings of this study correspond with that of a study conducted in New York concluded that approximately two-thirds of the healthcare facilities experience a shortage of staff and such staffing issues are associated with less timely immunisation delivery [23]. The findings are also similar to that of another study which alluded that nursing shortages are the main factor leading to errors, higher morbidity and mortality rates [24]. Furthermore, in clinical areas with high patient–nurse ratios, nurses experience burnout and dissatisfaction, [24].

4.1.2 Inadequate equipment and supplies

This study found that there is inadequate equipment and supplies such as cooler box and thermometer affects how cold chain is maintained during immunisation. This was confirmed by Participant 9 who said *'Okay, the challenges that we encounter we tend not to have portable fridge and then we are in a certain community and it far for the clinic we may find that the ice packs that we put in the cooler box tend to melt as such cold chain is broken'.*

Participant 10 also said *'The one challenge that I once experienced is that I was located in this clinic and the fridge was not properly working) to prepare and to put in the cooler box, the ice packs were not well iced and that is not good for the medication because they can spoil'.*

Participant 5 *'Sometimes the challenges that we would experience thermometer. sometimes they might not be working... so we just assume the temperature is correct even if we are not sure its correct or not'.*

The finding is supported by Mulatu et al. [25], who alluded that inappropriate handling of the vaccine and unavailability of the equipment all hurt the potency and efficacy of the vaccines used in immunisation. The absence of cold chain equipment due to faulty equipment was a challenge in more than a quarter of the health facilities and ensuring Extended Programme of Immunisation activities was a major concern. Electricity failure in urban and lack of gas in rural areas in a study conducted in Tanzania together with the absence of a contingency plan were the main challenges to the compliance with WHO temperature agreement in the storage of cold chain medicines in health facilities [16]. Furthermore, some of the health facilities were forced to keep their vaccines in other health facilities which is a challenge to travel before and after immunisation to collect and depot vaccines. Most cold rooms have insufficient storage capacity and incomplete equipment for adequate cold chain maintenance [16, 26].

4.1.3 Power supply interruption

In this study, it was revealed that power interruption such as load shading affect the functioning of the vaccine fridge, leading to the melting of ice pack, which interferes with cold chain maintenance.

Participant 12 stated that '*The challenge that I saw is that in the morning when we arrive, you will find that the fridge is off and ice packs were melting because of electricity, they said that the electricity went off during the night*'.

Participant 14: '*During power failure, there is a problem of backup for our fridges, vaccines are damaged*'.

The findings of this study are congruent with that of a study conducted in Mozambique which showed that the most common causes of power failure were flat batteries in solar refrigerators and improper adjustment of thermostats which affected the functioning of the refrigerator [27]. Similar findings were identified in a study conducted by [28] that elaborated that irregular power supply of health facilities, and the absence of standby generators are the major risk factors for loss of vaccine potency. The backup is a challenge as is in most developing countries and the shortage of power is one of the main causes of loss of cold chain maintenance since power outages are widespread concerns. Electricity failure in urban and lack of gas in rural areas in a study conducted in Tanzania together with the absence of a contingency plan were the main challenges to the compliance with WHO temperature agreement in the storage of cold chain medicines in health facilities [26]. Another study recommends the continuous control of temperature problems and equipment breakdowns through the introduction of temperature monitoring and control devices and best intervention practices [4].

4.2 Lack of knowledge and skills

The study findings revealed that there is a lack of knowledge and skills. The following sub-themes were identified, inadequate knowledge on cold chain maintenance, lack of in-service training on cold chain management and ignorance and negligence to adhere to cold chain principles.

4.2.1 Inadequate knowledge of cold chain maintenance

The finding of this study indicates that most nurses in the clinical area lack knowledge regarding the importance of maintaining a cold chain during immunisation. This leads to the mishandling and storage of vaccines which affects the maintenance of the cold chain.

This claim was supported by Participant 7 who stated, '*Challenges that are found during immunisation is that you may not be competent in withdrawing the content inside the vial and you that you take time holding the vial*'.

Participant 17 elaborated that '*Sometimes a nurse is allocated to monitor the temperature of the vaccine fridge and she does not check the temperature of the vaccine fridge twice daily, meaning that she will not know if the cold chain temperature is maintained in the fridge*'.

The findings are like that of a study by Pillay [29], who identified that specific staff members should be knowledgeable regarding vaccine storage and handling and there should be at least two healthcare workers who are responsible for vaccine management. The findings of this study indicated that negligence of the staff affects how nurses handle the vaccines and it may affect the maintenance of the cold chain. Vaccine cold chain management is suggestively associated with the overall cold chain management knowledge and profession of a healthcare worker in health institutions [15]. Most cold chain managers displayed inadequate knowledge while a significant number presented poor training in preserving the vaccines' cold chain [30].

4.2.2 Lack of in-service training on cold chain management

The study indicates that in-service training of health workers is important for maintaining a cold chain during immunisation. This claim was supported by Participant 3 who stated '*Mostly I think it is poor training. The nurses are not fully trained about the importance of maintaining cold chain which results in them holding the vaccine vials with their whole hand instead of holding them at the tip*'.

Participant 1 added '*They do not know how to pack the cooler box correctly and they just handle the vaccine anyhow and they put the cooler box directly on the floor whereby there is heat and they don't close the cooler box*'.

The study findings correspond with that of a study conducted by [31] which found that the vaccine cold chain issues is no longer simple, as new vaccines are added every day to the immunisation schedules and the responsible staff must be trained on different handling requirements. Training is required on temperature monitoring through new devices including electronic temperature recording monitors VVMS, as well as the use of cold ice packs. A study conducted in Southwest Burkina Faso stated that failure to maintain a safe temperature range by overheating freezing may lead to loss of vaccine potency. This can be caused by failure or inadequate staff training in temperature monitoring and fridge temperature adjustment [3]. Continuous in-service training and immunisation guidelines at work were recommended to improve health professionals' knowledge about a cold chain [10]. The provision of adequate cold chain management requires a pool of good knowledge amongst health professionals which appears much lower than the expected level indicating that there is a need to plan in-service- training for all people working with vaccines and those involved in the vaccination program [32].

4.2.3 Ignorance and negligence to adhere to cold chain principles

Ignorance and negligence of healthcare workers to the principles followed to maintain cold chain play an important role in immunisation to ensure the optimal potency of a vaccine, careful attention is needed in handling practice at all level of levels of the cold chain.

This was supported by Participant 11 who said, '*Sometimes in the morning you find that there is no ice in the refrigerator because it can be that the nurse who was immunising the previous day forgot to return the icepack in the refrigerator*'.

Participant 4 also *stated 'The stuff will still put food inside the fridge even though we discourage them, always opening the fridge to take their food therefore interfering with the cold chain'.*

Participant 15 added *'The challenge is that you might find that the vaccine fridge is not monitored, and we know that the temperature should be monitored daily'.*

The study indicates that sufficient knowledge is needed to maintain cold chain during immunisation and health workers whose work experience is more than two years were about five times more likely to have proper practice on cold chain management compared to their counterparts [25]. During the provision of immunisations in healthcare institutions, both doctors and nurses must share all information about the vaccination methods which includes making the cold supply chains stable rather than being negligent during patient care [33]. The study findings by [34] suggest providing empowerment and obstacle removal solutions to those forced to neglect and violate protocols for cold chain maintenance for various reasons are all essential elements of successful cold chain interventions [35]. Nurses who work in vaccination rooms should make efforts to prevent temperature changes and avoid losses and higher public expenses caused by their negligence and malpractice [34].

4.3 Suggestions to improve maintenance of cold chain

The participants in this study indicated some suggestions that they believe can improve the cold chain during immunisation at health facilities. Participants suggested the provision of adequate equipment for cold chain management, in-service training for nurses on cold chain management and the provision of a backup system for power interruptions.

4.3.1 Provision of adequate equipment for cold chain management

The study found that the provision of adequate equipment for cold chain management can improve the maintenance of the cold chain during immunisation in the clinical area.

Participant 3 stated *'If the nurses have problem with the infrastructure, they should report to the management so that the issues they are having such as not having air conditioners and having faulty cooler boxes can be fixed by the government'.*

Participant 16 stated that *'The government does not provide adequate or the renewal of vaccine fridge, which means that vaccines will be stored in refrigerators that store food because the vaccine fridge is broken, and the fridge will be opened frequently'.*

A study conducted in Cameroon stated that the absence of cold chain equipment in many health facilities ensuring EPI activities was a major preoccupation since these facilities are obligated to store their vaccines in other healthcare facilities which affected the maintenance of cold chain [28]. Almost 25% of health facilities were conducting EPI activities without cold chain equipment resulting in a threat to the cold chain for vaccines [29]. Effective cold chain management is not dependent on well-trained staff only but also relies on reliable cold chain equipment and temperature monitoring devices [36]. Correct vaccine storage and controlling of the cold chain method is fundamental for immunisation and to achieve this quality at the highest standard it requires adequate space, temperature monitoring and consistent defrosting with record keeping [37].

4.3.2 In-service training for nurses on cold chain management

This study found that the proper training of nurses in cold chain management can improve the maintenance of the cold chain during immunisation.

Participant 3 stated '*I think that nurses should be properly trained, like they should at workshop monthly where they are taught the importance of maintaining cold chain and how the immunisation process is done*'.

Participant 1 elaborated that '*They should do frequent in-service training to reduce ignorance with regard to maintenance of cold chain*'.

Participant 8 stated that '*In nursing schools they can teach student nurses how to maintain cold chain thoroughly so in detail*'.

Pre-service training is fundamental in the skills' acquisition of health care practitioners; however, they require additional in-service training and supportive supervision to function effectively in managing immunisation data tasks [38]. Similarly, a study conducted by [39] recommends continuous professional education and training for cold chain practitioners, to improve the maintenance of cold chain and improve monitoring and evaluation of cold chain activities [40] alluded that supervision alone appears to be not making a difference, but the provision of standardised in-service training, with practical demonstrations and well-designed regular supportive supervision is highly recommended. A study conducted by [41] indicated that many international studies have been conducted on the importance of in-service training and authors agree that in-service training improves the quality of nursing care. Training, supervision and monitoring of cold chain management were recommended as predictors of good cold chain management practices to be upheld by institutions [42]. The provision of regular technical support and on-the-job training on vaccine cold chain management is important to improve the knowledge, attitude and practice of vaccinators and vaccine handlers on proper maintenance of cold chain [43].

4.3.3 Provision of backup system for power interruptions

The findings of this study indicated that providing backup system for power interruptions in the clinic can improve the maintenance of cold chain.

Participant 9 stated '*I think maybe the department of health should try to bring backup generators in the health facilities, in the clinics so that it can act as a backup for electricity if there is load shedding for us to maintain cold chain*'.

Participant 3 stated '*I think since cold chain start in the fridge; they should make sure that the fridge works properly. if they have issues of electricity, they can put generators in case the electricity goes off*'.

The study findings correspond with that of a study conducted which recommends that the government should provide proper and adequate substitution for electricity in all the local government areas to ensure the cold chain is maintained continuously during electricity failure [44]. Furthermore, a backup system for power interruption such as the use of a generator or solar system is essential for the maintenance of the cold chain in healthcare facilities. Primary health care providers must ensure the availability of generators in case of power failure and proper management of vaccine fridges and cold chain boxes for effective cold chain for vaccines. Frequent cuts in the power supply can have a direct impact on storage temperature and the non-availability of standby generators will adversely affect vaccine potency at the vaccination centres. A possible device for the transition of Electric refrigerators with solar-derived refrigerators is required [40].

4.4 Conclusion

There are many challenges in the maintenance of cold chain in health care institutions that need immediate intervention to make cold chain a success. This chapter covered the introduction, the definition of concepts used in the chapter, the methodology employed in the chapter which relates to the research approach, the design, the population, the data collection and data analysis methods. The presentation, interpretation and discussion of the findings of the experiences of learner nurses concerning the maintenance of cold chain during immunisation from a university in Limpopo province, South Africa. Challenges such as a shortage of material resources, lack of knowledge and skills, and some suggestions to improve maintenance of the cold chain during immunisation were highlighted.

Acknowledgements

The authors would like to acknowledge the undergraduate student from a university in Limpopo province. South Africa who participated in the study.

Funding information

No funding was received for conducting the study.

Conflict of interest

The authors declare no conflict of interest.

Author details

Takalani Edith Mutshatshi* and Thabo Arthur Phukubye
University of Limpopo, Department of Nursing Science, Polokwane, South Africa

*Address all correspondence to: takalani.mutshatshi@ul.ac.za

IntechOpen

References

[1] Pambudi NA, Sarifudin A, Gandidi IM, Romadhon R. Vaccine cold chain management and cold storage technology to address the challenges of vaccination programs. Energy Reports. 2022;8:955-972

[2] South Africa Department of Health. Immunisation That Works: The vaccinator's Manual. 3rd ed. Pretoria: National department of health; 2015

[3] Sow C, Sanou C, Medah C, Schlumberger M, Mireux F, Ouédraogo I, et al. Challenges of cold chain quality for routine EPI in south-West Burkina-Faso: An assessment using automated temperature recording devices. Vaccine. 2018;36(26):3747-3755

[4] Ashok A, Brison M, LeTallec Y. Improving cold chain systems: Challenges and solutions. Vaccine. 2017;35(17):2217-2223

[5] World Health Organization. Study Protocol for Temperature Monitoring in the Vaccine Cold Chain. Geneva, Switzerland: World Health Organization; 2011. Available from: https://apps.who. int/iris/handle/10665/70752

[6] Shukla VV, Shah RC. Vaccinations in primary care. The Indian Journal of Pediatrics. 2018;85(12):1118-1127

[7] Nayir T, Nazlican E, Şahin M, Kara F, Meşe EA. Effects of immunization program on morbidity and mortality rates of vaccine-preventable diseases in Turkey. Turkish Journal of Medical Sciences. 2020;50(8):1909-1915

[8] Mugharbel KM, Al Wakeel SM. Evaluation of the availability of cold chain tools and an assessment of health workers practice in Dammam. Journal

of Family and Community Medicine. 2009;16(3):83-88

[9] Rahmat EG, Nita Y, Priyandani Y. The profile of cold chain management of vaccines in primary healthcare Centre in Kupang, Indonesia. Pharmacy Education. 2023;23(4):203-207

[10] Yassin ZJ, Yimer Nega H, Derseh BT, Sisay Yehuala Y, Dad AF. Knowledge of health professionals on cold chain management and associated factors in Ezha District, Gurage zone, Ethiopia. Scientifica. 2019;1:6937291

[11] Asamoah A. Knowledge, Attitude and Practice of Cold Chain Management Among Health Practitioners in the Sekyere Central District. 2020. (Doctoral Dissertation, University of Cape Coast)

[12] Asamoah A, Ebu Enyan NI, Diji AK, Domfeh C. Cold chain management by healthcare providers at a district in Ghana: A mixed methods study. BioMed Research International. 2021;2021(1):7559984

[13] World Health Organization. Immunization Supply Chain and Logistics: A Neglected but Essential System for National Immunization Programmes: A Call-to-Action for National Programmes and the Global Community by the WHO Immunization Practices Advisory Committee. Geneva, Switzerland: World Health Organization; 2014

[14] Syakur A, Sandra C, Bumi C. Evaluation of cold chain management. Journal management Kesehatan Indonesia. 2021;9(1):21-27. DOI: 10.14710/jmki.9.1.2021.21-27

[15] Ogboghodo EO, Omuemu VO, Odijie O, Odaman OJ. Cold chain management: An assessment of

knowledge and attitude of health workers in primary health-care facilities in Edo Etate Nigeria. Sahel Medical Journal. 2018;**21**(2):75-82. DOI: 10.4103/smj. smj_45_17

[16] Bogale HA, Amhare AF, Bogale AA. Assessment of factors affecting vaccine cold chain management practice in public health institutions in east Gojam zone of Amhara region. BMC Public Health. 2019;**19**(1):1433-1436. DOI: 10.1186/ s12889-019-7786-x_31675948

[17] Mothiba TM, Tladi FM. Challenges faced by professional nurses when implementing the expanded programme on immunisation at rural clinics in Capricorn District, Limpopo. African Journal of Primary Health Care and Family Medicine. 2016;**8**(2):1-5

[18] Republic of South Africa. The Nursing Act, Act No. 33 of 2005 as Amended. Pretoria: Government Printer; 13 March 2008

[19] Pham H, Wang H. Imperfect maintenance. European Journal of Operational Research. 1996;**94**(3):425-438. DOI: 10.1016/s0377-2217(96)00099-9

[20] Colapinto J. This is the Voice. New York, America: Simon and Schuster; 2021

[21] De Haan M, Dennhill K, Vasuthevan S. De Haan's Health of Southern Africa. In: Vasuthevan S, Mthembu S, editors. Johannesburg, South Africa: Juta; 2021

[22] de Beer H, Harmse J, Mielmann A. Why income lacks to ensure household food security: Needs and challenges identified by consumers from a rural community, South Africa. International Journal of Consumer Studies. 2020;**44**(6):521-530

[23] Grant, Turner NM, York DG, Goodyear-Smith F, Petousis-Harris HA.

Factors associated with immunization coverage and timeliness in New Zealand. British Journal of General Practice. 2010;**60**(572):e113-e120

[24] Alosaimi BB, Al-Dosari MM, Aldosari HM, Al Doseri AO, Alshammari KR, Almajdi T, et al. Nursing turnover-an overview and updates from kingdom of Saudi Arabia. Chelonian Research Foundation. 2022;**17**(2):2699-2709

[25] Mulatu S, Tesfa G, Dinku H. Assessment of factors affecting vaccine cold chain management practice in Bahir Dar City health institutions. American Journal of Life Sciences. 2020;**8**(5):107-113

[26] Ringo S, Mugoyela V, Kaale E, Sempombe J. Assessment of medicines cold chain storage conformity with the World Health Organization requirements in health facilities in Tanzania. Pharmacology and Pharmacy. 2017;**8**:325-338. DOI: 10.4236/ pp.2017.810024

[27] Lennon P, Atuhaire B, Yavari S, Sampath V, Mvundura M, Ramanathan N, et al. Root cause analysis underscores the importance of understanding, addressing, and communicating cold chain equipment failures to improve equipment performance. Vaccine. 2017;**35**(17):2198-2202

[28] Ateudjieu J, Kenfack B, Nkontchou BW, Demanou M. Program on immunization and cold chain monitoring: The status in eight health districts in Cameroon. BMC Research Notes. 2013;**6**(1):1-7

[29] Pillay S. A Descriptive Study into the Cold Chain Management of Childhood Vaccines by Nurses in Primary Health Care Clinics in the uMgungundlovu District (Doctoral dissertation)

[30] Feyisa D. Cold Chain Maintenance and Vaccine Stock Management Practices at Public Health Centers Providing Child Immunization Services in Jimma Zone in community health centers of Tikamgarh district of Madhya Pradesh. The International Journal of Community Medicine and Public Health. 2019;**6**(2):823

[31] Kartoglu Ü, Özgüler NK, Wolfson LJ, Kurzatkowski W. Validation of the shake test for detecting freeze damage to adsorbed vaccines. Bulletin of the World Health Organization. 2010;**88**:624-631

[32] Kasahun AW, Zewdie A, Mose A, Adane HA. Health professionals' knowledge on vaccine cold chain management and associated factors in Ethiopia: Systematic review and meta-analysis. PLoS One. 2023;**18**(11):e0293122

[33] Ahmed AA, Abouzid M, Eatmann AI. Vaccine: The Black Box. UK: Wellcome Trust, Independently Published; 2021

[34] Patine FD, Lourenção LG, Wysocki AD, Santos MD, Rodrigues IC, Vendramini SH. Analysis of vaccine loss due to temperature change. Revista Brasileira de Enfermagem. 2021;**74**(1):e20190762

[35] Rajabi-Arani Z, Asadi-Piri Z, Zamani-Alavijeh F, Mirhosseini F, Bigdeli S, Dandekar SP, et al. Examining the educational experiences of Behvarzes from the insufficient participation of some people in preventive measures against the COVID-19 pandemic: A lesson for the future. BMC Medical Education. 2024;**24**(1):785

[36] Kumar G, Gupta S. Assessment of cold chain equipments and their management in government health facilities in a district of Delhi: A cross-sectional descriptive study. Indian Journal of Public Health. 2020;**64**(1):22-26

[37] Panika RK, Prasad P, Nandeshwar S. Evaluation of vaccine storage and cold chain management practices during intensified mission Indradhanush

[38] Nicol E, Turawa E, Bonsu G. Pre-and in-service training of health care workers on immunization data management in LMICs: A scoping review. Human Resources for Health. 2019;**17**:1-4

[39] Erassa TE, Bachore BB, Faltamo WF, Molla S, Bogino EA. Vaccine cold chain management and associated factors in public health facilities and district health offices of Wolaita zone, Ethiopia. Journal of Multidisciplinary Healthcare. 2023;**16**:75-84

[40] Rogie B, Berhane Y, Bisrat F. Assessment of cold chain status for immunization in Central Ethiopia. Ethiopian Medical Journal. 2013;**51**(Suppl. 1):21-29

[41] Letlape HR, Koen MP, Coetzee SK, Koen V. The exploration of in-service training needs of psychiatric nurses. Health SA Gesondheid. 2014;**19**(1):1-9

[42] Eressa LA, Edossa TG. Lattice dynamical and thermodynamic properties study of ceria using density functional theory and Hubbard correction. Physica B: Condensed Matter. 2023;**651**:414600

[43] Mohammed SA, Workneh BD, Kahissay MH. Knowledge, attitude and practice of vaccinators and vaccine handlers on vaccine cold chain management in public health facilities, Ethiopia: Cross-sectional study. PLoS One. 2021;**16**(2):e0247459

[44] Ademuyiwa IY, Farotimi AA, Owopetu CA, Olaogun AA, Oyeleye AB. Challenges in the maintenance of cold chain system: A case study of IFE-Desha zones of Osun state, Nigeria. West African Journal of Nursing. 2017;**28**(1):85-91

Chapter 5

Transforming Primary Care Practice through Strategic Reform in the Republic of Srpska

Darijana Antonić and Slobodan Stanić

Abstract

The development of the healthcare system in former Yugoslavia and Bosnia and Herzegovina began in the twentieth century, between 1919 and 1937. Another significant period in the system's development occurred after the Second World War and during the reform of primary care from 1976 to 1992, which aimed to establish family medicine clinics in primary care. After the civil war, Bosnia and Herzegovina (B&H) split into two entities, the Republic of Srpska and the Federation of B&H, along with the Brčko District. Under the Constitution of the Republic of Srpska, the Republic of Srpska possesses all state functions and jurisdictions, with limited international subjectivity. The Ministry of Healthcare and Social Welfare in the Government of the Republic of Srpska assumed full responsibility for the functioning of the healthcare system within the Republic of Srpska. This chapter aims to present strategic directions for transforming primary care, with a particular focus on family medicine in the Republic of Srpska. We will use a framework approach consisting of three complex levels: structure, process, and outcomes, with each level measuring several dimensions of primary care.

Keywords: reform, primary care, family medicine, structure, process, outcomes

1. Introduction

The Republic of Srpska's commitment to reform processes in primary healthcare is reflected in several reform documents that influenced the drafting of new amendments to existing legal regulations regarding the reorganisation of primary healthcare, specifically the organisation of this care according to the family medicine model. Family medicine represents a different approach to primary healthcare by focusing on the continuous preservation and improvement of the population's health, with the patient, family and community at the centre.

The first Law on Healthcare was adopted in 1993, which began to define a new way of organising and functioning the health system in general, as well as primary healthcare, in the Republic of Srpska [1].

According to the 1993 Law, the health centre (dom zdravlja) became the basic form of organising primary healthcare. It is carried out according to the principles of unified healthcare and teamwork, utilising dispensary and social-medical methods, which also provides the conditions for implementing primary healthcare for the whole family. By defining the health centre's role in this way, the preconditions for the primary healthcare reform process were established, resulting in the adoption in 1996 of the Strategy for the Development of Healthcare in the Republic of Srpska by the Year 2000, which was created based on the principles of the World Health Organisation's strategy 'Health for All by the Year 2000' [2].

The Strategy for the Development of Healthcare in the Republic of Srpska by the Year 2000, in chapter IV, 'Development of the Healthcare and Health Insurance System', identifies as one of its goals the reorientation of the existing primary healthcare, with an emphasis on solving the majority of health problems through the implementation of promotional, preventive and curative measures and rehabilitation, all with the active support of individuals, families and the community.

The Strategy for the Development of Healthcare in the Republic of Srpska by the Year 2000 served as the foundation for creating a strategic document: the Strategic Plan for the Reform and Reconstruction of the Health System 1997–2000 [3]. This document also places the reorganisation of primary healthcare according to the family medicine model at the centre of the reform process. The reorganisation of primary healthcare did not diminish the importance of health centres within the healthcare system, as their role remains vital in providing consultative-specialist services (such as paediatrics and gynaecology) and diagnostic-laboratory support for the services delivered by family medicine teams.

The 1999 Law on Healthcare was a reform law that, among other provisions, mandated that health centres, as primary healthcare institutions, be organised according to the family medicine system [4]. Based on this legal framework, the family medicine team became the first point of contact for citizens entering the healthcare system. Organising according to the family medicine model means that the family medicine team provides healthcare for all family members and takes responsibility for the health of the community in which it operates. The proponents of the Law on Healthcare were guided by international standards regarding the organisation of primary healthcare, that is, the definition of family medicine given by the Regional Office of the World Health Organisation (WHO) for Europe (1998). According to this definition, family medicine is at the centre of the health system, emphasising the effectiveness of family medicine as 'general, continuous, comprehensive, coordinated, collaborative healthcare oriented to the family and the immediate community [5]. In this regard, special emphasis is placed on the rational use of health resources in the health system, both in the vertical hierarchy and in the horizontal activity when using diagnostic and other technical means'. With the adoption of this Law, preconditions were created for the introduction of the concept of family medicine in the Republic of Srpska. The introduction of this concept was supported by the Basic Health Project (BHP) from 2000 to 2004, during which the following activities were carried out:

1. Demonstrating the concept of family medicine in pilot regions in the Republic of Srpska (health centres Laktaši, Čelinac, Doboj and Banjaluka) and the Federation of Bosnia and Herzegovina,

2. Providing support for accompanying medical education (further education in family medicine for doctors' other specialities),

3. Focusing on financing and managing the health sector.

The family medicine model was successfully established and tested in the mentioned health centres.

The experiences gained during the implementation of the project 'Basic Healthcare' served as the basis for adopting the Primary Healthcare Strategy, which defined the strategic goals for developing primary healthcare in the Republic of Srpska over a five-year period (2006–2010) [6]. The project 'Strengthening the Health Sector', financed by the World Bank and the Council of Europe Development Bank, supported the implementation of the Strategy's goals. Achieving the fundamental strategic goal, strengthening the position of primary healthcare in the healthcare system of the Republic of Srpska and expanding the family medicine model to all health centres in the Republic of Srpska entailed amendments to the existing legal regulations. The Law on Healthcare adopted in 2009 [7] and amendments adopted in 2015 [8], served as the basis for drafting new and refining existing by-laws. The Law preserves the basic concept of primary healthcare while promoting the centrality of the family medicine model and focusing on health promotion, prevention, suppression and early detection of diseases, treatment and rehabilitation.

The organisational reform of the health system in the Republic of Srpska was simultaneously accompanied by the reform of the financing of mandatory health insurance institutions with the adoption of the Law on Health Insurance in 1999 with changing and added [9]. This Acts, which refers to financing health institutions from compulsory health insurance, is harmonised with the new way of organising primary healthcare based on the family medicine model.

2. The context of the Republic of Srpska

2.1 The Republic of Srpska and population

The Dayton Peace Agreement was signed on 13 December 1995. According to Article 1 of the Dayton Agreement and the Constitution of Bosnia and Herzegovina, Bosnia and Herzegovina is a country that consists of two Entities (the Republic of Srpska and the Federation of Bosnia and Herzegovina) and the Brčko District. Based on this agreement and the Constitution of the Republic of Srpska, the Republic of Srpska, one of the entities in Bosnia and Herzegovina, has all state functions and competencies and limited international subjectivity. The Republic of Srpska has an area of 24,641 km^2 (49% of the territory of Bosnia and Herzegovina) with a population density of 59 inhabitants per km^2, thus belonging to the group of sparsely populated regions. According to estimates from the Institute of Statistics, the Republic of Srpska has about 1.1 million inhabitants, of which about 49% are men and 51% are women. Of the age groups, about 13% of the inhabitants are aged 0–14, about 68% 15–64, and 19% are aged 65+ [10].

2.2 Development and economy

Gross domestic product (GDP, nominal) in 2022 was about 14.54 billion convertible marks (KM) (EUR 7.5 billion), with a real growth rate of 3.9% compared with 2021. GDP per capita is KM 11,080 (EUR 5682). The unemployment rate has shown a downward trend in the last few years (14.30% in 2021 and 11.20% in 2022) [11].

The total expenditures of the Health Insurance Fund of the Republic of Srpska for mandatory health insurance amounted to over 800 million KM (2017) and 1.1 billion

KM (2023), while the expenditures of the Health Insurance Fund of the Republic of Srpska for primary healthcare amounted to approximately 230 million KM (2017) [12] and 280 million (2023) [13]. The total number of insured persons was 913,275 (2017) and 930,167 (2023). That is, about 80% of the citizens of the Republic of Srpska had the right to use healthcare from mandatory health insurance.

2.3 Populations' health

In the Republic of Srpska, as in most European countries, chronic non-communicable diseases, such as cardiovascular diseases, malignant diseases and endocrine gland disorders (diabetes), dominate the morbidity and mortality of the population. The average age of those who died in 2018 was 74.45 years, and 74.83 years in 2022. The birth rate is about eight live births per 1000 inhabitants. The natural increase shows a negative trend due to the higher number of deaths compared to the number of live births [10].

3. The context of primary healthcare

Primary healthcare is a subsystem of the overall health system. Its specific characteristic is that well-organised primary healthcare contributes to easy access to and use of coordinated health services by a country's population. To examine primary healthcare in the Republic of Srpska, we used the primary healthcare framework, observed through ten dimensions grouped into three categories (structure, processes and outcomes) [14].

3.1 Structure and organisation of primary healthcare

3.1.1 Managing of the primary healthcare

The adoption of the five-year Primary Healthcare Strategy (2006–2010) was aimed at laying the foundations for the functioning of primary healthcare based on the family medicine model. This involved amendments to existing legislation to establish more efficient and financially stable primary healthcare.

The healthcare system of the Republic of Srpska is relatively centralised because the Ministry of Health and Social Welfare in the Government of the Republic of Srpska (hereafter: the Ministry) is responsible for planning public health institutions, ensuring equal access and ensuring patients' rights. Likewise, the Ministry is responsible for strategic planning through the development and implementation of health policies and the creation of the planning framework, and all key administrative and regulatory functions are under the competence of this Ministry. The government is the founder of health institutions at the secondary and tertiary levels, and institutions have a particular form of public health organisation (Institute for Public Health). The Ministry is responsible for planning and overseeing capital investments in health institutions. The Ministry has four departments, one of which is the Healthcare Department, which has a dedicated Department of Primary Healthcare.

The relatively centralised role of the Ministry is primarily reflected in the fact that the local self-government (cities and municipalities) is responsible for establishing health centres as an institution at the primary level of healthcare. In addition to the role of the founder, local self-government in accordance with the provisions of the

Law on Healthcare also has certain responsibilities regarding the organisation and operation of primary healthcare [15].

The last Decision on the plan of the network of health institutions does not comply with the new Law of Healthcare [16]. The criteria defined in the now invalid Decision refer to the number of inhabitants (insured persons) per family medicine team and the distance of the family medicine clinic from the farthest household (8 km). Those two criteria are insufficient to define the exact number of family medicine teams, that is, to ensure equal availability of family medicine services. The plan for the network of family medicine ambulances specifies the number of family medicine ambulances in the public network in each local self-government. This may contribute to the continued dominance of family medicine teams in public ownership in the Republic of Srpska.

In the Republic of Srpska, no overall allocations for primary healthcare are planned because health centres can be financed from different sources and each source (Health Insurance Fund of the Republic of Srpska, Government of the Republic of Srpska and local self-government) plans these needs in its budget, and in addition to these sources, institutions can be financed from other sources prescribed in accordance with current legislation.

Inspection work in the healthcare field is under the competence of the Health Inspection of the Republic of Srpska. There is no separate department that deals with matters of supervision of the work of institutions at the primary level of healthcare.

In the Republic of Srpska, no special law deals with patients' rights, but the Law on Healthcare defines all patients' rights. One of the fundamental human rights guaranteed by this Law is the right to healthcare, which manifests through the right to choose a doctor of family medicine freely, information regarding one's health, then the right to inspect medical documentation, freely choose medical treatment and consent to it. Protection of the rights of insured persons from compulsory health insurance is defined by special regulations adopted by the Health Insurance Fund of the Republic of Srpska [17].

Regarding establishing health institutions, the Rulebook on the conditions for starting the operation of health institutions was adopted, which prescribes the minimum requirements in terms of personnel, space and equipment necessary for establishing a health institution [18]. According to the Law on Healthcare, public and private institutions in the Republic of Srpska are established under the same conditions. The participation of privately owned healthcare institutions has been increasing in recent years, and the most represented institutions at the primary level of healthcare are pharmacies and dental clinics. Private healthcare institutions also provide primary healthcare services, with private specialist family medicine clinics being less represented than other primary-level institutions (dental clinics, pharmacies).

The number of privately owned institutions (specialist clinics and specialist centres) at the secondary level of healthcare has been increasing since the Health Insurance Fund of the Republic of Srpska offered the possibility of signing contracts with specialists in a particular branch of medicine (paediatricians, gynaecologists, ophthalmologists, dermatologists), to provide more accessible healthcare in rural areas.

3.1.2 Economic situation in primary healthcare

Healthcare in the Republic of Srpska is primarily financed by mandatory health insurance, with the Health Insurance Fund of the Republic of Srpska acting as the purchaser of health services in the mandatory health insurance system. The Health Insurance Fund of the Republic of Srpska is funded from various sources, and the most important source of income of the Health Insurance Fund of the Republic of Srpska (over 80%) is funds collected based on contributions for mandatory health insurance. The Health Insurance Fund of the Republic of Srpska covers the costs of primary, secondary and tertiary healthcare for insured persons, as well as the costs of purchasing medicines, transportation to hospital treatment, medical equipment and benefits for sick leave over 30 days. The Health Insurance Fund contracts with both public and private health institutions.

The Health Insured Fund of the Republic of Srpska contracts the provision of primary health care services with health centres for the provision of family medicine, consultative and specialist services (paediatrics and gynaecology), diagnostics (laboratory, radiology and ultrasound), dentistry, hygiene and epidemiological services, protection and improvement of mental health, community rehabilitation and emergency medical care. The services provided by the family medicine team are contracted for all insured persons covered by that health centre; individual contracts are not concluded with each family medicine team within the health centre. Employees in the family medicine team are paid according to the Law on Salaries of Persons Employed in Public Institutions in the Health Sector of the Republic of Srpska [19].

One of the reasons for the reform of primary healthcare was related to the inefficiency of the provision of health services, which is a consequence of high expenditures in healthcare and the emphasis on secondary and tertiary healthcare. In the Republic of Srpska, inefficient provision of health services is still evident because the data of the Health Insurance Fund of the Republic of Srpska for secondary and tertiary care are continuously increasing. Therefore, the emphasis is still placed on secondary and tertiary healthcare at the expense of primary healthcare.

The Health Insurance Fund of the Republic of Srpska uses different criteria to determine the amount of compensation for providing primary healthcare services (normative staffing in the work team and the number of insured persons or the number of citizens per work team). Family medicine services for insured persons over the age of 6 are paid according to the capitation model, while the amount of funds is determined based on two parameters, general capitation and weighted capitation coefficient, by age group [20]. The principles, conditions and criteria for concluding contracts with public and private health service providers are prescribed by the Health Insurance Fund of the Republic of Srpska annually. The Health Insurance Fund of the Republic of Srpska enters into a contract for family medicine services for insured persons with health centres and private health institutions, including privately owned institutions. The content of the services provided in family medicine relates to health promotion, disease prevention, curative healthcare, home treatment and prescribing medications, with the noted Rulebook not defining the scope and content of the services provided in the basic package of health services for family medicine.

3.1.3 Employees in family medicine teams

A team consisting of a family medicine specialist (team leader) and two nurses provides family medicine services.

At the time of the transition to the concept of family medicine, to ensure a sufficient number of family medicine doctors, all doctors employed in health centres at that time were allowed to complete further education in family medicine. Today, family medicine doctors acquire the title of specialist in family medicine upon completion of a 36-month specialisation in family medicine.

The title of specialist in family medicine is awarded by the Faculty of Medicine in Banja Luka and the Faculty of Medicine in Foča. After completing their specialisation in family medicine, doctors are obliged to complete continuous education and regularly renew their licences with the Chamber of Doctors of Medicine of the Republic of Srpska. Doctors of family medicine established their professional association—the Association of Doctors of Family Medicine of the Republic of Srpska, which contributes to creating guidelines for good practice in family medicine. Given that the process of implementing family medicine in the Republic of Srpska is still not fully completed and that the process of educating the required number of specialists in family medicine could not be realised by the end of 2030, jobs in family medicine may currently be performed by doctors, specialists in other branches of medicine, with additional education about family medicine practice [15].

Nurses/technicians employed in the family medicine team must also have education in family medicine or acquire it within the same time frame, that is, until the final implementation of the family medicine model.

4. Providing family medicine services

4.1 Access to family medicine doctors

Ensuring an adequate number of family medicine doctors is a prerequisite for the availability of family medicine services. In the Republic of Srpska, there is no strategy for human resources; therefore, there is no defined national standard for the number of family medicine doctors. The analysis of the required number of specialisations/subspecialisations from all branches of medicine, including specialists in family medicine, is conducted by the Public Health Institute of the Republic of Srpska to meet the needs of the Ministry. The analysis and planning of the necessary staff in family medicine, based only on the criteria prescribed by the Rulebook on the Basic Standards and Norms of Healthcare from the mandatory health insurance, does not fully reflect the actual needs for the number of family medicine doctors or other members of the family medicine team [21]. Criteria defined by this Rulebook include insured persons for whom one work team provides family medicine activities or the average annual number of visits (5.4 visits) of the entire work team (doctor and nurses) per insured person. The number of insured persons depends on the development of local self-government (from 600 insured persons in undeveloped and extremely undeveloped to 2000 insured persons in developed self-government).

In the Republic of Srpska, the total number of doctors of family medicine employed in health centres in 2022 was 630, of which 400 were specialists in family medicine or specialists in another branch of medicine, with additional education in family medicine, 44 doctors specialising in family medicine and 186 doctors without specialisation [22]. Also, privately owned family medicine teams (about 30) provide family medicine services in medicine clinics or specialist care centers.

4.2 Access to family medicine services

The family medicine team provides family medicine services during eight-hour working days, or 40 hours a week. Outside the working hours of the family medicine team, emergency medical centres provide healthcare services. Specialist family medicine clinics do not belong to institutions that are obliged to provide 24-hour healthcare to registered/insured patients. However, in exceptional cases, the Health Insurance Fund of the Republic of Srpska may contract a specialist family medicine clinic to provide 24-hour healthcare.

4.3 The way providing family medicine teams services

Family medicine teams schedule registered patients for an examination.

Family medicine services are primarily provided through direct contact between the patient and the doctor and, to a lesser extent, telephone consultations. In 2022, family medicine doctors had an average of about 130 visits (first and follow-up visits) per week with patients in the clinic [22].

Also, the family medicine team organises and conducts treatment in the insured person's home when such treatment is justified and medically necessary, that is, in cases where the sick and injured cannot use outpatient services due to their health condition. In 2022, family medicine teams performed 250,636 home visits, with family medicine doctors performing 16,985 home visits and 233,651 by nurses/technicians [22].

4.4 Financial barriers in family medicine

The financing of the right to healthcare for insured persons is provided in full by the Health Insured Fund of the Republic of Srpska using mandatory health insurance funds, with the participation of the insured persons in the costs (co-payment). The Health Insured Fund of the Republic of Srpska determines the amount of co-payment for providing family medicine services. Insured patients pay a co-payment ranging from 1.00 to 1.50 KM for each visit to the doctor of family medicine, regardless of whether it is an examination by a doctor of family medicine or prescription medicine or a referral to another specialist or hospital treatment. Co-payments for home visits are slightly higher than those for outpatient clinic examinations. The amount is determined by the distance of the family medicine outpatient clinic from the place of residence of the insured person (up to 5 km is 1.8 KM, and over 5 km is 4.5 KM). Likewise, the Health Insured Fund of the Republic of Srpska has defined the categories of insured persons exempt from co-payments for healthcare costs [17].

Charges for other services provided within the scope of work by family medicine team members are applied to insured persons according to the valid pricelist of the Health Insurance Fund of the Republic of Srpska.

Uninsured persons are required to pay the total amount for health services provided by family medicine based on the valid pricelist of the Health Insurance Fund of the Republic of Srpska. Furthermore, the insured person has the right to reimbursement of healthcare costs in cases where they have paid for healthcare costs for justified or unjustified reasons.

4.5 Continuity of family medicine services

Citizens of the Republic of Srpska are guaranteed by law the right to choose a doctor of family medicine freely. Insured persons opt for a family medicine doctor for one year, after which they can choose another family doctor or stay with the same one. The choice is made according to the place of residence and, in exceptional cases, also outside the place of residence to ensure more accessible and efficient healthcare. This right can be challenged only if the family doctor has reached the maximum number of certain insured persons and if there are strained interpersonal relations between the insured person and the family doctor.

The family medicine doctor refers insured persons to diagnostic procedures (laboratory, radiological and other tests), consultative specialist examinations and hospital treatment, that is, to institutions that have signed a contract with the Health Insurance Fund of the Republic of Srpska. The referral is accompanied by documents and findings collected at the primary level of healthcare, and family medicine receives feedback on the health status of the referred insured person in the form of findings/opinions and a discharge letter.

According to the Law on Health Documentation and Record in the Field of Healthcare, the family doctor is obliged to open the health record at the first contact with the patient, keep records of each contact and deliver the health record to another family doctor, in the event of a change of family doctor or a change of the patient's place of residence [23]. Health records are kept in electronic form, and until 2019, there was not a single database of electronic patient records because different electronic platforms (Dr Medic and Web Medic) were used to manage electronic records. Since 2020, family medicine doctors have used a unique database (the Integrated Health Information System of the Republic of Srpska). Family medicine teams use this electronic database for prescribing medications, issuing referrals, checking the patient's insurance status (insured or not), and sometimes for electronic communication with the laboratory diagnostic service.

4.6 Coordination of family medicine services

In the Republic of Srpska, the role of family medicine doctors as gatekeepers is partially realised because patients can request and receive some health services without being referred to by family medicine doctors. This includes consultative-specialist services of gynaecologists (primary level of healthcare) for women over 15 years of age, paediatricians and dental healthcare in public or private healthcare institutions. Similarly, patients can also use the services of other specialists who work in privately owned healthcare institutions without a family medicine doctor's instruction, though in that case, they fully bear the costs of healthcare.

With the introduction of the family medicine model, in addition to the doctor of family medicine, the work team includes two nurses, and the role of the nurse has remained unchanged. In the Republic of Srpska, there are no special teaching programs for the specialised education of nurses to provide services at the primary level of healthcare within the health sciences faculties. Likewise, there is no legal framework for establishing the Chamber of Nurses as an organisational structure that would licence nurses, which is why nurses participate minimally in continuous medical education. In this regard, no association of primary healthcare nurses focuses narrowly on the issues and problems of providing nurses' services in primary healthcare.

In the Republic of Srpska, all health institutions, including the family medicine teams, have a legal obligation to submit individual or collective reports in paper/tabular form for the use of healthcare services and the health status of the population using those services and information about human resources to the Public Health Institute of the Republic of Srpska twice a year (semi-annually/annually).

They must submit individual reports in written form (report of malignant neo-plasm, report of infectious disease, etc.) to the Public Health Institute of the Republic of Srpska once the disease has been diagnosed. The information in these two types of reports enables the Public Health Institute of the Republic of Srpska to analyse the population's health status annually. In contrast, other data from the patient's health records are used rarely to identify the population's health needs at the local and regional levels or to define health policy priorities related to primary healthcare.

4.7 Comprehensiveness of family medicine services

Family medicine clinics, in addition to the staff necessary to start work, have a legal obligation to meet the requirements regarding equipment, which allows them to provide a wide range of health services, including diagnosing acute conditions, monitoring chronic conditions and diseases, promoting healthy lifestyle habits and preventing many risk factors for mass non-communicable diseases.

5. Outcomes of family medicine services

5.1 Quality and safety of providing family medicine services

The Republic of Srpska is committed to providing safe and high-quality health services by adopting the 'Policy for Improving the Quality and Safety of Healthcare in the Republic of Srpska until 2010' [24]. One of the strategic goals of this Policy was the definition and adoption of the legal framework to strengthen the structure and process of establishing and improving the safety and quality of healthcare. This strategic goal was achieved in 2009 by adopting the Law on Healthcare and introducing voluntary accreditation and mandatory certification of health institutions.

The determination to improve the quality of healthcare is indicated by one of the objectives of the Primary Healthcare Strategy, which refers to the introduction and application of quality standards to improve, ensure and control healthcare quality [6]. To monitor and evaluate the metrics of healthcare quality and safety indicators, the Ministry previously adopted the Rulebook on Monitoring the Quality of Work in Healthcare Institutions [25], and then the new Rulebook on Quality Indicators, including the way of monitoring and evaluating the quality and safety of health-care in healthcare institutions [26]. An integral part of the Rulebook includes indica-tors of the quality of work of primary healthcare, that is, indicators of the quality of work of the specialist clinic-team of family medicine. Monitoring and evaluating these indicators is the responsibility of the Agency for Certification, Accreditation and Improvement of Healthcare Quality of the Republic of Srpska. Since 2007, the Rulebook has been adopted, but the Agency has yet to fully establish a system for monitoring indicators in all specialist clinics/family medicine teams.

5.2 Effectiveness of providing family medicine services

The existing system for monitoring the efficiency of work and the provision of family medicine services is not fully effective because, according to the Primary Healthcare Strategy, the creation of a Strategy for Monitoring and Evaluation of the

Health System of the Republic of Srpska [6] was necessary to develop and implement the monitoring and evaluation system. This Strategy would ensure that all organisational forms at the primary healthcare level, including family medicine clinics, continuously collect data based on indicators for systematic monitoring and evaluation. Also, using defined indicators, progress would be monitored in terms of short-term, medium-term and long-term goals defined by the framework of health policies, strategies, programs and projects. The Public Health Institute of the Republic of Srpska should play a key role key in implementing these activities.

Likewise, there are no official indicators of patient satisfaction regarding various aspects of using family medicine services, nor indicators for measuring employees' satisfaction in family medicine. These could be a significant source of information for health policymakers in defining further goals for developing family medicine.

6. Conclusion

The healthcare system of Bosnia and Herzegovina was an integral part of the healthcare system of the Socialist Federal Republic of Yugoslavia. After the breakup of Yugoslavia and the civil war in Bosnia and Herzegovina, three independent health systems began to function in Bosnia and Herzegovina (healthcare systems of the Republic of Srpska, Federation of Bosnia and Herzegovina and Brčko District).

The Republic of Srpska thus began the transformation of all segments of its health system, including primary health care, which represents the entry point into the health system. The fundamental basis for the reform of primary health care and the transition to the family medicine model was initiated by the Reform Law on Health Care in 1999.

The reform process of primary healthcare in the Republic of Srpska developed a new way of organising it using the family medicine model. It has passed its critical period of stabilising and functioning primary healthcare; however, in the coming period, it is necessary to take specific measures toward more innovative financing of family medicine teams through payment for the scope and quality of service provision. It is also essential to innovate ways of paying doctors and nurses in the family medicine team to stimulate younger doctors to stay at the primary level of health care. It is also necessary to promote entrepreneurial initiatives among family medicine teams that function as part of health centres in the direction of functioning of as many teams as independent health institutions. All the mentioned measures and activities would lead to long-term stability and solve numerous upcoming problems in primary health care.

Author details

Darijana Antonić[1]* and Slobodan Stanić[2]

1 Public Health Institute of the Republic of Srpska, Pan-European University "Apeiron" Banja Luka, Banja Luka, The Republic of Srpska, Bosnia and Herzegovina

2 Public Health Institute of the Republic of Srpska, Faculty of Pharmacy and Health, University of Travnik, Banja Luka, The Republic of Srpska, Bosnia and Herzegovina

*Address all correspondence to: darijana.a@gmail.com

IntechOpen

References

[1] Narodna skupština Republike Srpske. Zakon o zdravstvenoj zaštiti [Law on healthcare]. Službeni Glasnik Republike Srpske. 1993;**II**(12):472-481

[2] Narodna skupština Republike Srpske. Strategija razvoja zdravstvene zaštite u Republici Srpskoj do 2000. godine [Strategy for the Development of Healthcare in the Republic of Srpska by the Year 2000] 1996

[3] Ministartsvo zdravlja i socijalne zaštite Republike Srpske. Strateški plan za reformu i rekonstrukciju zdravstvenog sistema 1997-2000 [Plan for the Reform and Reconstruction of the Health System 1997-2000] 1997

[4] Narodna skupština Republike Srpske. Zakon o zdravstvenoj zaštiti [Law on healthcare]. Službeni Glasnik Republike Srpske. 1999;**VIII**(18):367-374

[5] Svjetska zdravstvena organizacija - Regionalni ured za Evropu. Okvir za profesionalni i administartivni razvoj opće prakse/obiteljske medicine u Evropi. EUR/HFA, Target 28, Copanhagen, 1998

[6] Radna grupa projekta Evropske unije/Svjetske zdravstvene organizacije "Podrška reformi zdravstvene zaštite u Bosni i Hercegovini 2004-2006." Strategija primarne zdravstvene zaštite [Primary Healthcare Strategy], Banja Luka, 2008

[7] Narodna skupština Republike Srpske. Zakon o zdravstvenoj zaštiti [Law on healthcare]. Službeni Glasnik Republike Srpske. 2009;**XVIII**(106):1-16

[8] Narodna skupština Republike Srpske. Zakon o izmjenama i dopunama zakona o zdravstvenoj zaštiti [Law on amendments to the law on health care].

Službeni Glasnik Republike Srpske. 2015;**XXIV**(44):17-18

[9] Narodna skupština Republike Srpske. Zakon o zdravstvenom osiguranju [Law on health insurance]. Službeni Glasnik Republike Srpske. 1999;**VIII**(18):360-367

[10] Repunlički zavod za statistiku Republike Srpske. Demografska statistika, 2023 [Demographic Statistic, 2023], Banja Luka, 2023

[11] Investiciono-razvojna banka Republike Srpske. Baza podataka o ekonomskim indikatorima Republike Srpske - IRBRS. Available from: https://www.irbrs.net/statistika/UporedniPrikaz.aspx?tab=3&lang=lat [Accessed: August 20, 2024]

[12] Službeni glasnik Republike Srpske. Saopštenje o ukupnim izdacima za zdravstveno osiguranje Fonda za zdravstveno osiguranje Republike Srpske za 2017. godinu [Announcement on the Total Expenditures for Health Insurance of the Health Insurance Fund of the Republic of Srpska for the Year 2017], Broj: 82/18, 2018

[13] Fond zdravstvenog osiguranja Republike Srpske. Saopštenje o ukupnim izdacima za zdravstveno osiguranje Fonda za zdravstveno osiguranje Republike Srpske za 2023. godinu [Announcement on the Total Expenditures for Health Insurance of the Health Insurance Fund of the Republic of Srpska for the Year 2023], Broj: 02/002/2656-7-1/24, 2024

[14] Kringos DS, Boerma WG, Hutchinson A, van der Zee J, Groenewegen PP. The breadth of primary care: A systematic literature review of its core dimensions. BMC Health Services Research. 2010;**10**(1):1-13

[15] Narodna skupština Republike Srpske. Zakon o zdravstvenoj zaštiti Republike Srpske [Law on healthcare]. Službeni Glasnik Republike Srpske. 2022;**XXXI**(1-42):15-16

[16] Vlada Republike Srpske. Odluka o planu mreže zdravstvenih ustanova [Decision on the plan of the network of health institutions]. Službeni Glasnik Republike Srpske. 2001;**X**(2):13-15

[17] Narodna skupština Republike Srpske. Zakon o obaveznom zdravstvenom osiguranju [Law on compulsory health insurance]. Službeni Glasnik Republike Srpske. 2022;**XXXI**(93):1-22

[18] Ministarstvo zdravlja i socijalne zaštite Republike Spske. Pravilnik o uslovima za početak rada zdravstvenih ustanova. Službeni Glasnik Republike Srpske. 2017;**XXVI**(53):6-80

[19] Narodna skupština Republike Srpske. Zakon o platama zaposlenih lica u javnim ustanovama u oblasti zdravstva Republike Srpske [Law on salaries of persons employed in public institutions in the health sector of the republic of Srpska]. Službeni Glasnik Republike Srpske. 2022;**XXXI**(68):3-7

[20] Fond zdravstvenog osiguranja Republike Srpske. Pravilnik o osnovima za zaključivanje ugovora sa davaocima zdravstvenih usluga u Republici Srpskoj za 2024. godinu [Rulebook on the basis for concluding contracts with health service providers in the Republic of Srpska for the year 2024]. Službeni Glasnik Republike Srpske. 2023;**XXXII**(111):35-69

[21] Fond zdravstvenog osiguranja Republike Srpske. Pravilnik o osnovama standarda i normativa zdravstvene zaštite iz obaveznog zdravstvenog osiguranja [Rulebook on the basics of health care standards and norms from compulsory health insurance]. Službeni Glasnik Republike Srpske. 2024;**XXXIII**(48):6-26

[22] Šiljak S, Štrkić D, Rodić Vukmir N, Petković V, Todorović M. Zdravstveno Stanje stanovništva [Health Status of the Population]. Banja Luka: JZU Institut za javno zdravstvo, Republika Srpska [Public Health Institute, Republic of Srpska]; 2022

[23] Narodna skupština Republike Srpske. Zakon o zdravstvenoj dokumentaciji i evidencijama u oblasti zdravstva [Law on health documentation and records in the field of health]. Službeni Glasnik Republike Srpske. 2022;**XXXI**(57):44-45

[24] Radna grupa Vlade Republike Srpske. Politika unapređivanja kvaliteta i sigurnosti zdravstvene zaštite u Republici Srpskoj do 2010 [Policy for Improving the Quality and Safety of Health Care in the Republic of Srpska Until 2010], Banja Luka, 2010

[25] Ministartsvo zdravlja i socijalne zaštite Republike Srpske. Pravilnik o praćenju kvalitetu rada u zdravstvenim ustanovama [Rulebook on monitoring the quality of work in healthcare institutions]. Službeni Glasnik Republike Srpske. 2007;**XVI**(74):7-12

[26] Ministartsvo zdravlja i socijalne zaštite Republike Srpske. Pravilnik o indikatorima kvaliteta, načinu praćenja i evaluacije kvaliteta i sigurnosti zdravstvene zaštite u zdravstvenim ustanovama [Rulebook on quality indicators, methods of monitoring and evaluating the quality and safety of healthcare in healthcare institutions]. Službeni Glasnik Republike Srpske. 2019;**XXIX**(59):15-19

www.ingramcontent.com/pod-product-compliance
Lightning Source LLC
Chambersburg PA
CBHW081242190326
41458CB00016B/5888